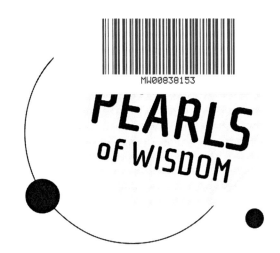

PEARLS
of WISDOM

Occupational and Environmental Medicine
REVIEW

Michael I. Greenberg, M.D., M.P.H.

McGraw-Hill
Medical Publishing Division

New York Chicago San Francisco Lisbon London
Madrid Mexico City Milan New Delhi
San Juan Seoul Singapore
Sydney Toronto

Occupational and Environmental Medicine Review

Copyright © 2006 by The McGraw-Hill Companies, Inc. All rights reserved. Printed in the United States of America. Except as permitted under the United States Copyright Act of 1976, no part of this publication may be reproduced or distributed in any form or by any means, or stored in a data base or retrieval system, without the prior written permission of the publisher.

1 2 3 4 5 6 7 8 9 0   CUS/CUS   0 9 8 7 6 5

ISBN 0-07-146438-7

Notice

Medicine is an ever-changing science. As new research and clinical experience broaden our knowledge, changes in treatment and drug therapy are required. The authors and the publisher of this work have checked with sources believed to be reliable in their efforts to provide information that is complete and generally in accord with the standards accepted at the time of publication. However, in view of the possibility of human error or changes in medical sciences, neither the authors nor the publisher nor any other party who has been involved in the preparation or publication of this work warrants that the information contained herein is in every respect accurate or complete, and they disclaim all responsibility for any errors or omissions or for the results obtained from use of the information contained in this work. Readers are encouraged to confirm the information contained herein with other sources. For example and in particular, readers are advised to check the product information sheet included in the package of each drug they plan to administer to be certain that the information contained in this work is accurate and that changes have not been made in the recommended dose or in the contraindications for administration. This recommendation is of particular importance in connection with new or infrequently used drugs.

The editors were Catherine A. Johnson and Marsha Loeb.
The production supervisor was Phil Galea.
The cover designer was Handel Low.
Von Hoffmann Graphics was printer and binder.

This book is printed on acid-free paper.

Cataloging-in-Publication data for this title is on file at the Library of Congress.

INTERNATIONAL EDITION ISBN: 0-07-110877-7

Copyright © 2006. Exclusive rights by The McGraw-Hill Companies, Inc. for manufacture and export. This book cannot be re-exported from the country to which it is consigned by McGraw-Hill. The International Edition is not available in North America.

INTRODUCTION

Congratulations! *Occupational and Environmental Medicine Review: Pearls of Wisdom*, will help you improve your knowledge base in medicine. Originally designed as a study aid to improve performance on the Boards exam, this book is full of useful information. A few words are appropriate in discussing intent, format, limitations and use.

Since *Occupational and Environmental Medicine Review* is primarily intended as a study aid, the text is written in a rapid-fire question/answer format. This way, readers receive immediate gratification. Moreover, misleading or confusing "foils" are not provided. This eliminates the risk of erroneously assimilating an incorrect piece of information that makes a big impression. Questions themselves often contain a "pearl" intended to reinforce the answer. Additional "hooks" may be attached to the answer in various forms, including mnemonics, visual imagery, repetition, and humor. Additional information, not requested in the question, may be included in the answer. Emphasis has been placed on distilling trivia and key facts that are easily overlooked, quickly forgotten and that somehow seem to be needed on board examinations.

Many questions have answers without explanations. This enhances ease of reading and rate of learning. Explanations may often occur in a later question/answer. Upon reading an answer, the reader may think, "Hm, why is that?" or "Are you sure?" If this happens to you, go check! Truly assimilating these disparate facts into a framework of knowledge absolutely requires further reading of the surrounding concepts. Information learned in response to seeking an answer to a particular question is retained much better than information that is passively observed. Take advantage of this! Use this book with your preferred texts handy and open.

Occupational and Environmental Medicine Review risks accuracy by aggressively pruning complex concepts down to the simplest kernel—the dynamic knowledge base and clinical practice of medicine is not like that! Furthermore, new research and practice occasionally deviates from that which likely represents the right answer for test purposes. This text is designed to maximize your score on a test. Refer to your most current sources of information and mentors for direction for practice.

Occupational and Environmental Medicine Review is also designed to be re-used several times to allow memorization. A hollow bullet is provided for any scheme of keeping track of questions answered correctly or incorrectly.

We welcome your comments, suggestions and criticism. Great effort has been made to verify these questions and answers. Some answers may not be the answer you would prefer. Most often this is attributable to variance between original sources. Please make us aware of any errors you find. We hope to make continuous improvements and would greatly appreciate any input with regard to format, organization, content, presentation, or about specific questions.

Study hard and good luck!

MIG

TABLE OF CONTENTS

OCCUPATIONAL MEDICINE

INDUSTRIAL HYGIENE ASPECTS FOR THE OCCUPATIONAL PHYSICIAN.................................11

OCCUPATIONAL TOXICOLOGY 19

LEAD...25

MERCURY 31

CADIUM 37

SOLVENTS...41

CHEMICAL CARCINOGENESIS 47

WORKPLACE DRUG TESTING..55

ERGONOMICS 63

CARPAL TUNNEL SYNDROME 69

NOISE..73

VIBRATION 81

OCCUPATIONAL RELATED CANCER..85

OCCUPATIONAL EPIDEMIOLOGY 91

STATISTICS...101

SILICOSIS..111

TRAUMATIC EMERGENCIES 119

MUSCULOSKELETAL...139

IONIZING RADIATION 149

OCCUPATIONAL RELATED INFECTIOUS DISEASES 165

WORKERS' COMPENSATION...183

OCCUPATIONAL RELATED HEMATOLOGICAL PROBLEMS 191

OCCUPATIONAL RELATED HEPATIC PROBLEMS..199

OCCUPATIONAL RELATED RENAL PROBLEMS...207

REGULATORY ISSUES..215

ENVIRONMENTAL MEDICINE

HEAT-RELATED ILLNESS..235

ALTITUDE-RELATED ILLNESS 243

UNDERSEA MEDICINE 251

BITES AND STINGS...259 N/A

COLD-RELATED MEDICAL PROBLEMS 267

ENVIRONMENTAL DISASTERS...279

WATER POLLUTION...285

OUTDOOR AIR POLLUTION 293

WEAPONS OF MASS DESTRUCTION 301

MASS-CASUALTY WEAPONS I: GENERAL, TOXINS AND RADIATION 305

MASS-CASUALTY WEAPONS II: BIOLOGICAL AGENTS 319

MASS-CASUALTY WEAPONS III: CHEMICAL AGENTS 331

BIBLIOGRAPHY 347

OCCUPATIONAL MEDICINE

INDUSTRIAL HYGIENE ASPECTS FOR THE OCCUPATIONAL PHYSICIAN

❍ **What is Industrial Hygiene?**

The health profession devoted to the recognition, evaluation and control of occupational and environmental hazards.

❍ **How does a fume differ from a smoke?**

Fumes contain particles usually less than 1 micron, while smoke particles are less than 0.1 microns and are usually produced by incomplete combustion of carbonaceous materials.

❍ **The estimated average cost of each employee injury/accident is approximately?**

$20,000.

❍ **OSHA fines are the result of violations involved in employee accidents is set at a maximum of _____ for each egregious and/or flagrant violation.**

$70,000.

❍ **What are the four major elements that make up a basic safety and health program?**

Management, commitment, and employee involvement; work site hazards analysis, hazard prevention and control, and safety and health training.

❍ **As part of work site hazard analysis all recognize hazards are those hazards that are _____ to the work being performed.**

Typical.

❍ **Usually in America (men, women and children, young and old) how many will have an injury so severe that they will lose a day of work or school or go to a hospital or physician for treatment due to an accident at work, at home, traveling, or at play at school?**

1 in 3.

○ **The OSHA hazard communication standard requires what 5 components?**

Written hazard communication program, maintain a list of all hazardous chemicals in the workplace, available MSDS, container labels, worker education, and training.

○ **The most commonly used heavy-duty abrasive for metal surfaces are _____?**

Silica sand, metal shot, slags, or silicon carbide.

○ **Name three major types of blasting used to deliver abrasives in the workplace.**

Pressure blasting, hydroblasting, centrifugal wheel blasting.

○ **Name the two main types of degreasing processes.**

Cold decreasing, vapor decreasing.

○ **Retroplating is done to provide what properties to either metal, plastic or rubber?**

Appearance, to reduce electrical resistance, to provide electrical insulation, a base for soldering or to improve wear ability.

○ **Name seven common plating metals used in electroplating processes.**

Cadmium, chromium, copper, gold, nickel, silver and zinc.

○ **Approximately how many workers are involved in electroplating in the U.S.?**

160,000.

○ **Name five grinding wheel abrasives.**

Aluminum oxide, silicon carbide, natural diamonds, synthetic diamonds, cubic boron nitride.

○ **Vibration white finger syndrome has been associated with what grinding techniques?**

Portable grinders and pedestal mounted wheel grinders.

○ **It has been estimated that _____ cases of dermatitis occur each year from contact with coolants and cutting fluids?**

400,000.

○ **Soluble oils frequently cause what type of dermatitis?**

Eczematous.

○ **Straight oils (insoluble) cutting fluids cause what type of dermatitis?**

Folliculitis

○ **Cutting fluid coolant sampling techniques exist for determination of contamination by what substances?**

Bacteria, yeast, and fungi.

○ **The characteristic smell of a machine shop is related to what?**

Oil mist from hot cutting fluids.

○ **Name the three main types of cutting fluids.**

Mineral oil, emulsified oils, and synthetics.

○ **Mineral oil base is composed of what percentages of paraffinic or naphthenic oils?**

60-100%.

○ **Emulsified oil (soluble oil) is an opaque milky-appearing mineral oil that is typically diluted with water to what ratio?**

1:5 – 1:50.

○ **Synthetic cutting oils are comprised of what percent water?**

50-80%.

○ **Conventional paint is an inorganic pigment dispersed in a vehicle, which also consists of _____?**

Binder, solvent, selected fillers and additives.

○ **Describe the two-part drying process of conventional varnishes.**

Evaporation of the solvent followed by oxidation of the resin binder, pigmented varnish.

○ **Pigmented varnish is also known as _____?**

Enamel.

○ **Give five examples of white pigments included in paints.**

Bentonite, kaolin clay, talc, titanium dioxide and zinc oxide.

○ **Give several examples of extenders used to control viscosity in paints.**

Talc, clay, calcium carbonate, barite, and silica.

○ **Pigments and extenders represent a potential hazard during what process?**

Sanding, or surface preparation.

○ **Name four fungicides that have been included in paints.**

Copper, zinc naphthenate, copper oxide, and Tributyltin oxide.

○ **Waterborne paints represent what % of construction industry paints?**

15-20%.

○ **What are the favorable properties of epoxy paint systems?**

Adhesive properties, resistance to abrasions and chemicals, and stability at high temperatures.

○ **Describe the process of soft soldering.**

Joining of metal by surface adhesion without melting the base metal. Tarnishes frequent component of metals, must be removed during the soldering and braising processes.

○ **Name three causes for tarnish.**

Oxides, sulfides, and carbonates.

○ **Flux is designed to remove what from a base metal surface until a solder is applied?**

Absorb gases and tarnish.

○ **Resin, a common base for organic fluxes contains what acid as the active material?**

Abietic acid.

○ **Describe the three major flux bases.**

Inorganic, organic non-resin, organic resin.

○ **Why are organic non-resins favored during the soldering process?**

They are less corrosive and slower acting and do not present the handling hazards that inorganic acids do.

○ **Solder generally contains what percent of metals?**

65% tin and 35% lead.

○ **Traces of other metals are commonly found in solder and they include___?**

Cadmium, bismuth, copper, iron, aluminum, nickel, zinc.

○ **The number of special solders may contain antimony concentrations up to ___?**

5%.

○ **In general, how many types of common flux materials are there?**

10.

○ **How is braising different from soldering?**

Braising is defined as a technique for joining metals that are heated above 800° F, whereas soldering is conducted below 800° F.

○ **Shielded metal arc welding is also commonly called ____?**

Stick or electrode welding.

○ **Describe electric arc welding.**

An electric arc is established between the welding rod and the work piece melting the metal along the seam or surface.

○ **Most commonly DC voltages of 10-50 are used at a wide range of currents. What is the upper amperage that is commonly used in DC arc welding?**

2000.

○ **Shielded metal arc welding has the potential to produce what?**

Nitrogen oxides which tend not to exceed 0.5 ppm under normal operating conditions.

○ **What are other names for gas tungsten arc welding?**

Tungsten inert gas, heliarc welding.

○ **Gas tungsten arc welding technique is routinely used for welding materials such as _____?**

Aluminum and magnesium, stainless steel, nickel alloys, brasses, silver, bronze.

○ **Inert gas technique of welding introduced welders to what type of electromagnetic radiation?**

UVB ultraviolet B light.

○ **The use of personal protective equipment (PPE) makes the most sense when?**

The hazard cannot be fully controlled by using other means.

○ **Why should personal protective equipment be viewed as an organization/line of defense?**

It takes significant effort by the organization to ensure that proper PPE is worn in every instance.

○ **What is the possible negative impact of wearing hearing protective devices?**

Placing these on already hearing impaired workers might make them less able to hear background warning sounds.

○ **What is the most important factor in determining whether or not PPE will be worn?**

User comfort.

○ **What are the main characteristics important in the selection of chemical protective clothing?**

Permeation, degradation, and penetration.

○ **Based on EPA personal protective ensembles, describe Level Protection A.**

Pressure demand full-face SCBA in a fully encapsulating chemical-resistant suit, which includes gloves and shoes, 2-way communication.

○ **Based on EPA personal protective ensembles, describe Level Protection B.**

Pressure demand full-face SCBA, chemical-resistant clothing over all, long-sleeved jacket, hooded. One or two-piece chemical splash suit or disposable chemical-resistant suit including boots and gloves, hardhat and two-way communication.

○ **Based on EPA personal protective ensembles, describe Level Protection C.**

Full-face air purifying canister equipped with respirator, chemical-resistant clothing including boots and gloves, two-way radio communication.

O **Based on EPA personal protective ensembles, describe Level Protection D.**

Coveralls, safety boots and shoes, safety glasses or chemical splash goggles, hardhat.

O **According to the American National Standards Institute (ANSI) hard hats are categorized in three classes. Describe Class A.**

Provides protection against impact and exposure to low voltage conductors, proof tested at 2200 volts and has a full brim.

O **According to the American National Standards Institute (ANSI) hard hats are categorized in three classes. Describe Class B.**

Baseball cap-like bill that protrudes out over the wearer's eyes, providing full protection against impact and exposure to high voltage conductors, proof tested at 20,000 volts.

O **According to the American National Standards Institute (ANSI) hard hats are categorized in three classes. Describe Class C.**

Provides protection against impact only, finds use especially in the forestry industry.

O **How is a BUMP different than a hardhat class C?**

BUMP caps are thin-shelled caps with a front bill worn for strike against hazards in the environment in areas of low head room. They are not designed for protection against falling objects.

O **Why is it recommended that contact lenses be worn with safety glasses or goggles?**

Contact lenses are considered to offer no protectin to the eye from any hazards because of partial coverage of the eye by contact lenses.

O **What is the leading cause of worker fatality in the U.S.?**

Falls from heights.

O **Approximately how many people are injured and killed from falls from heights?**

150-200 workers are killed annually with more than 100,000 injured.

O **Describe a personal fall arrest system used for fall protection.**

Limit the maximum resting force in a worker to 900 pounds with a body belt or 1800 pounds with a body harness, to be released that a worker may free fall no more than six feet nor contact with any lower level.

○ **According to the ANSI what is the color code for air purifying HEPA filters?**

Purple.

○ **The biological exposure indices (BEI) is an indicator of what?**

Uptake of a substance in the body.

○ **What does BEI generally indicate?**

A concentration below which nearly all workers should not experience adverse health effects.

○ **Air monitoring to determine TLV indicates what?**

Potential inhalation exposure of an individual or a group.

○ **Most BEIs are based on a direct correlation with what?**

The TLV-TWA and the concentration of the determinant, which can be expected when the airborne exposure is at the TLV-TWA.

○ **Regarding urine specimen acceptability for BEI testing, what guidelines are indicated for acceptable specimens?**

Creatinine concentration greater than 0.3 g/L and < 3.0 g/L or a specific gravity >1.010 and < 1.030.

OCCUPATIONAL TOXICOLOGY

❍ **Chronic, low-level, exposure to vinyl chloride may put a worker at risk for what cancer?**

Angiosarcoma of the liver.

❍ **What is green-leaf tobacco sickness?**

Found in tobacco harvesters who pick leaves by hand without gloves. Absorption of the nicotine from the dew-laden leaves leads to nausea, vomiting, headache, pallor, dizziness and diaphoresis.

❍ **Silo filler's disease is caused by high concentrations of what chemical?**

Nitrogen dioxide, NO_2.

❍ **What malignancy can be related to asbestos exposure?**

Mesothelioma.

❍ **What percent of mesotheliomas are probably due to asbestos exposure?**

Anywhere from 20 to 50% of mesotheliomas occur in individuals with no known asbestos exposure.

❍ **What are the two main groups of asbestos fiber?**

Ampibole and Chrysotile.

❍ **What is the OSHA PEL for manganese?**

5 mg/m^3.

❍ **What is the primary route of exposure for occupational lead exposure?**

Inhalation.

❍ **Manure pits emanate what toxic gases?**

Hydrogen sulfide, methane.

❍ **Which form of asbestos has been most commonly used in construction in the USA?**

Chrysotile.

O   **Chronic toxicity from what substance is often misdiagnosed as sarcoidosis?**

Berrylium.

O   **Arsine gas exposure can result in what hematologic problem?**

Hemolysis.

O   **What is metal fume fever?**

Headache, shortness of breath, chest pain and fever in a patient who has been exposed to heated metal, particularly cadmium and zinc.

O   **What is the treatment of metal fume fever?**

Mainly supportive with analgesics and antipyretics. Patients with metal fume fever generally do not have significant absorption. However, patients with pneumonitis or pulmonary edema should have levels checked.

O   **What is the blood lead level where a worker must be removed from occupational lead exposure according to OSHA standards?**

50ug/Dl.

O   **What is the current OSHA standard for airborne asbestos in the workplace?**

0.2 fibers / cc of air as an 8-hour TWA.

O   **What is the latent period between time-of-exposure to asbestos and lung cancer?**

10-30 years or more.

O   **What substance is responsible for chloracne?** *(molar/pre-auricular areas)*

Polychlorinated biphenyls (PCBs) as well as hexachlorodibenzo-p-dioxin, poylbrominated *compounds* dibenzofurans and biphenyls, polychlorinated dibenzofurans and tetrachloroazobenzene.

O   **Workers who fumigate fruits and vegetables at US ports of entry may be exposed to what chemical?**

Methyl bromide.

O   **What is degreasers flush?**

A disulfiram type reaction associated with alcohol intake following trichloroethylene exposures.

○   **What is the primary mission for NIOSH?**

NIOSH's primary mission is research.

○   **What does "OSHA" stand for?**

Occupational Health and Safety Administration.

○   **Which agency originally promulgated the Biologic Exposure Index (BEI)?**

ACGIH.

○   **What chemical is metabolized in the human body into carbon monoxide?**

Methylene chloride.

○   **What renowned legal matter allowed female workers to be exposed even though they could be pregnant?**

UAW versus Johnson Controls.

○   **What documents are required to be kept on site where dangerous industrial chemicals are found?**

Material Safety data Sheet (MSDS).

○   **Chloracne is associated with exposure to what toxic materials?**

Polychloirinated/polybromiated compounds.

○   **On what part of the body is chloracne most frequently found?**

Malar eminances and pre-auricular area.

○   **Which hydrocarbon, in the occupational setting, has been associated with the development of peripheral neuropathy?**

N-hexane.

○   **How does exposure to Portland cement cause skin burns?**

When water is added to cement powder calcium oxalate solution with a pH of approximately 13 results. This can cause a caustic skin burn the appearance of which may be delayed up to 24 hours.

❍   **Occupational exposure to vinyl chloride has been associated with what unusual bony abnormality?**

Acro-osteolysis.

❍   **What is Stoddard Solvent?**

A petroleum distillate that contains both aliphatic and aromatic hydrocarbons. It is also known as Varnoline, Varsol, and white spirits.

❍   **What is the most common occupationally related skin toxin?**

Poison ivy.

❍   **What is TSCA?**

The Toxic Substances Control Act; allows the EPA to obtain data from industry regarding the use, production and health effects of chemicals.

❍   **What toxic material is responsible for the most occupationally related toxic deaths each year?**

Carbon monoxide.

❍   **What toxic material is responsible for the second most occupationally related toxic deaths?**

Hydrogen sulfide.

❍   **Occupational exposure to benzidine is associated with the development of which cancer?**

Bladder.

❍   **Occupational exposure to chromium compounds is associated with the development of which cancer?**

Lung, nasal cavity.

❍   **Occupational exposure to coke oven emissions is associated with the development of which cancer?**

Bladder, lung, skin

❍   **What percent of all cancers can be attributed to occupationally based exposures?**

2-8%.

❍   **What is byssinosis?**

A pulmonary syndrome associated with occupational exposure to cotton and hemp.

❍   **What is characteristic of incidents wherein workers succumb to hydrogen sulfide?**

Multiple deaths; typically well meaning rescuers without proper protective equipment.

❍   **What is the treatment for hydrogen sulfide casualties?**

Removal from exposure, immediate administration of oxygen, prompt administration of thiosulfate as in cyanide poisoning, possible sue of hyperbaric oxygen.

❍   **What is "PPE"?**

Personal Protective Equipment.

❍   **Occupational exposure to what nematocide has been associated with oligospermia in male workers?**

Dibromochloropropane (DBCP).

❍   **The "Intermediate syndrome" is associated with exposure to what chemicals?**

Organophosphate pesticides.

❍   **Exposure to what industrial chemical may produce a green tongue?**

Vanadium.

❍   **What characterizes the toxic mechanism of action of the wood preservative pentachlorophenol?**

Uncoupling of oxidative phosphorylation producing a hypermetabolic state.

LEAD

○ **How many workers are exposed to lead every year in the United States?**

1 million.

○ **What is the most important route of absorption in occupational lead exposure?**

Inhalation.

○ **What size of lead particles increases the risk of inhalational absorption?**

< 5 um.

○ **Which occupations are at highest risk of worker lead toxicity?**

Ship breaking, welders, smelters, battery manufacturers/recycler/repairers, crystal glassmakers, polyvinyl chloride manufacturers, firing range employees, and construction workers (removal of lead paint).

○ **What percentage of inhaled lead is absorbed?**

30-40%.

○ **What percentage of ingested lead is absorbed in adults?**

10-15%.

○ **What percentage of ingested lead is absorbed in children?**

40-50%.

○ **What factors increase gastrointestinal absorption?**

Fasting/starvation and deficiencies in iron, zinc and cadmium.

○ **Does lead cross the placenta?**

Yes.

○ **What percentage of absorbed lead is immediately bound to erythrocytes?**

99%.

○ **What percentage of total body lead is stored in bone in an adult?**

95%.

○ **What are the three stages of lead distribution in the body?**

Lead is absorbed and immediately is bound to RBCs (the RBC pool), then it distributes to the soft-tissue (the soft-tissue pool) and, finally, to the more stable bone compartment (the bone pool).

○ **Is lead absorbed through the skin?**

The alkyl lead compounds, such as tetraethyl lead, are lipid soluble and readily absorbed through intact skin.

○ **What are the main two pathophysiologic effects of lead on cellular systems?**

Lead binds to electron-donating sulfhydryl groups and impacts numerous enzyme systems. Lead also is chemically similar to calcium and can interfere with calcium-related metabolic pathways, such as protein kinase.

○ **What is a "Burton line" or a "lead line"?**

A purple-blue line on the gingiva of people exposed to lead. The line consists of precipitated lead sulfide.

○ **What are the effects of acute lead toxicity?**

Encephalopathy, headache, and gastrointestinal cramping.

○ **What is the mechanism of encephalopathy induced by lead?**

Lead alters calcium cellular effects resulting in separation of intercellular junctions and capillary leak. Lead also alters neurotransmitter function.

○ **What are the effects of chronic lead toxicity?**

Anemia, headache, gastrointestinal cramping, peripheral neuropathy, renal insufficiency, hypertension and reduction in sperm counts and mobility.

○ **What type of neuropathy is induced by lead?**

A predominantly motor neuropathy may occur.

○ **What is the mechanism of neuropathy in lead toxicity?**

Lead-induced neuropathy develops initially from Schwann cell destruction, followed by demyelination and axonal degeneration.

O   **What is the mechanism of lead-induced anemia?**

Lead shortens the RBC lifespan by inhibiting Na/K ATPase and pyrimidine-5-nucleotidase. Lead also inhibits hemoglobin production by inhibition of several enzymes.

O   **What is "saturnine gout"?**

The association between working with lead and gout noted by the English physician Garrod.

O   **Why does lead exposure increase a worker's risk of gout?**

Lead inhibits the excretion of uric acid.

O   **What is "lead colic"?**

The crampy abdominal pain, nausea, vomiting and constipation associated with lead toxicity.

O   **At approximately what blood lead level does hemoglobin synthesis decrease in adults?**

50 micrograms/dL.

O   **Approximately what blood lead level is associated with increased risk of nephropathy?**

40 micrograms/dL.

O   **Approximately what blood lead level is associated with increased risk of hypertension in men?**

30 micrograms/dL.

O   **What are the typical symptoms of tetraethyl lead toxicity?**

Nausea, vomiting, tremor and encephalopathy. The organic lead compounds cause less hematologic manifestations than inorganic lead compounds.

O   **According to OSHA, what action should be taken for a worker with a routine blood lead screening concentration of 60 micrograms/dL?**

Immediate removal from worksite and a repeat blood lead level every month.

O   **When can a worker, who was removed from the worksite because of an elevated blood lead level, return to the worksite?**

When the blood lead level has returned to below 40 micrograms/dL.

O   **According to OSHA, what action should be taken for a worker with a routine blood lead screening concentration of 50 micrograms/dL?**

If a blood lead level between 40-60 micrograms/dL is found on a routine screen, then the worker must receive a repeat blood lead level in 2 months.

O   **What is the treatment of an adult or child with lead-induced encephalopathy?**

BAL 75 mg/m^2 every 4 hours for 5 days and CaNa EDTA 1500 mg/m^2/d as continuous infusion or divided q2-4 hours.

O   **What is the treatment of an adult worker with mild symptoms of lead toxicity?**

Oral succimer 350 mg/m^2 TID for 5 days, then BID for 14 days.

O   **What is the treatment of an asymptomatic adult worker with a blood lead concentration of 70-100 micrograms/dL?**

Oral succimer 350 mg/m^2 TID for 5 days, then BID for 14 days.

O   **What is the most important action in decreasing lead's toxicity?**

Removal from the source of lead or protecting the worker from continued exposure.

O   **How is smoking at the work place connected to lead toxicity?**

Smoking encourages hand-to-mouth behavior. Eating and drinking in the workplace have a similar effect.

O   **What is the half-life of lead in the bony compartment?**

25 years.

O   **Can this lead be mobilized back into the circulation?**

Yes, during stress, pregnancy, lactation, chronic disease or, possibly, osteoporosis.

O   **What characteristic finding may be seen on microscopic examination of the RBC in patients with chronic led toxicity?**

Basophilic stippling.

O **What three substances accumulate secondary to lead's inhibition of heme synthesis?**

Delta-aminolevulinic acid, coproporphyrinogen, and erythrocyte protoporphyrin.

O **BAL cannot be given to patients with what allergy?**

Peanuts.

O **In what group of patients must BAL be given cautiously?**

Those with G6PD deficiency.

O **What trace element deficiency can develop with CaNaEDTA chelation for lead?**

Zinc.

O **What percentage of total body lead is chelated in a typical course of chelation therapy?**

1-2%.

O **Why is BAL started prior to CaNaEDTA in encephalopathic lead toxic patients?**

Because CaNaEDTA may displace lead from tissues into the brain and worsen encephalopathy. This phenomena has been demonstrated in rats, but not in humans.

O **What are the characteristic microscopic findings of lead-induced renal damage?**

Nuclear inclusion bodies in renal tubular cells that are composed of a lead-protein complex.

O **What enzymes in the hemoglobin synthesis pathway are inhibited by lead?**

Delta ALA dehydratase, ALA synthetase, coproporphyrinogen decarboxylase, and ferochelatase.

O **In what foods might significant lead concentrations be found?**

"Moonshine" whiskey, calcium supplements, lead-foil covered wine, and canned foods (pre 1991 in the US or imported cans) from cans with lead solder.

O **Are lead paints still used in the United States?**

Household use of lead-based paint was stopped in 1978, however, lead-based paint is still used on ships and in non-household settings.

MERCURY

○ **What are the three forms of mercury?**

Elemental, inorganic and organic.

○ **Is elemental mercury absorbed in the GI tract?**

No. Ingestion of elemental mercury does not result in toxicity unless damage to the GI tract (e.g. fistula or perforation) is present.

○ **What is the primary route of absorption of elemental mercury?**

Inhalation. _via vaporization_

○ **What factors increase vaporization of elemental mercury and, therefore, inhalation?**

Aerosolization (as when the mercury is vacuumed) or heating.

○ **What percentage of an inhalational elemental mercury exposure is absorbed?**

75-80%.

○ **What is the primary route of absorption of inorganic and organic mercury?**

Both are primarily absorbed via the GI tract, but can be absorbed dermally.

○ **What percentage of inorganic mercury is absorbed in the GI tract?**

10%.

○ **What percentage of organic mercury is absorbed in the GI tract?**

90%.

○ **Long-chain and aryl organic mercury compounds produce toxicity that is most similar to organic or inorganic mercury?**

Inorganic mercury. The long chain and aryl groups are cleaved shortly after absorption to produce inorganic mercuric ion.

○ **Elemental mercury concentrates in what organ(s)?**

CNS and kidney.

O   **Inorganic mercury concentrates in what organ(s)?**

Kidney.

(Organic)

O   **Methyl mercury concentrates in what organ(s)?**

CNS and RBCs.

O   **Which forms of mercury are easily transferred across the placenta?**

(Organic)

Short-chain organic compounds, like methyl mercury.

(Organic)

O   **What is the major route of elimination of methyl mercury?**

Fecal.

O   **What is mercury's biochemical effect that causes toxicity?**

Mercury covalently binds to sulfur thereby inhibiting multiple enzymes and transport systems.

O   **What is the clinical toxicity of inhaled elemental mercury?**

Interstitial pneumonitis, pulmonary fibrosis, as well as tremor and renal dysfunction.

O   **What is the acute toxicity of inorganic mercury?**

Gastroenteritis and acute tubular necrosis.

O   **What is the chronic toxicity of inorganic mercury?**

Gingivostomatitis, gastroenteritis, tremor, fatigue, depression, "shyness", ataxia, constriction of visual fields ("tunnel vision"), proteinuria, and nephritic syndrome.

O   **What is "pink disease"?**

An idiosyncratic hypersensitivity to mercury that leads to erythematous, edematous, hyperkeratotic lesions on the hands, face and feet. The rash eventually leads to desquamation. Other symptoms include sweating, tachycardia, anorexia, tremors, paresthesias, insomnia and weakness.

O   **What kind of mercury is thimerosal?**

Thimerosal is a long-chain alkyl mercury compound.

Mercury compound

O   **Where is thimerosal found?**

Thimerosal is used as a bacteriostatic agent in vaccines and other IM shots.

O   **What is the toxicity of short-chain organic mercury compounds?**

Toxicity is almost entirely CNS including tremors, ataxia, hyperreflexia, movement disorders, and paresthesias.

O   **What is the toxicity found in children whose mothers were exposed to methyl mercury?**

Developmental delay, deafness, blindness, seizures and spasticity.

O   **What laboratory test is helpful in determining a mercury exposure?**

Urine 24 hour mercury.

O   **What is the treatment for acute moderate to severe inorganic mercury toxicity?**

BAL and DMSA.

O   **What is the toxicity of chronic inhalation of elemental mercury?**

It is similar to inorganic mercury toxicity; tremor, gingivostomatitis, and movement disorders.

O   **Does elemental mercury cross the blood brain barrier?**

Yes.

O   **How does elemental mercury produce CNS toxicity?**

Elemental mercury is oxidized to inorganic mercuric ion which then binds sulfur groups.

O   **What is erethism?**

Shyness, withdrawal, depression, irritability and frequent blushing that is associated with chronic mercury exposure.

O   **Is there mercury in dental amalgam?**

Yes.

O   **Does dental amalgam cause exposure to elemental mercury?**

Yes, approximately 1.5-10 ug/day.

○   **Is there any evidence that dental amalgam causes and clinical effects?**

No.

○   **Which form of mercury is a stool fixative, used in containers for ova and parasites?**

Mercuric chloride (inorganic mercury).

○   **Do any of the mercury compounds produce any caustic burns?**

Yes, inorganic mercury salts, e.g. mercuric chloride, may produce oral or gastrointestinal caustic burns if ingested.

○   **What is Minamata Disease?**

A factory dumped inorganic mercury into Minamata Bay. The fish converted inorganic mercury to organic mercury and when the human inhabitants of the area around Minamata Bay ingested the fish, they developed organic mercury toxicity, called Minamata disease.

○   **Which forms of mercury can be detected in urine?**

Elemental and inorganic. (methyl) Organic mercury is excreted mostly in the feces.

○   **What is the urinary half-life of inorganic mercury?**

Approximately 40 days.

○   **What is the blood half-life of inorganic mercury?**

Approximately 3 days.

○   **What test can detect long-term mercury exposure?**

Urine can detect chronic exposure. In addition, hair testing can detect mercury exposure over a longer period, but may be contaminated by environmental mercury.

○   **What oral chelators are available to chelate mercury?**

DMSA and d-penicillamine.

○   **What are the "Danbury shakes"?**

Mercury induced tremor seen in felt hat-makers in Danbury, CT.

○   **How is mercury used in hat production?**

Mercury nitrate was used to mat animal fur to make the felt.

○   **Is BAL indicated for all mercury toxicities?**

No, BAL is not indicated in organic mercury toxicity.

○   **What is quicksilver?**

Elemental mercury (Hg0).

○   **In what occupations are workers at risk of <u>elemental mercury</u> exposure?**

Production of amalgam, barometers, thermometers, paint, paper pulp and dentists, electroplaters, jewelers, photographers and mercury refiners.

○   **In what occupations are workers at risk of <u>inorganic mercury</u> salt exposure?**

Manufacturing of dyes, disinfectants, explosives, fireworks, vinyl chloride and tanners, laboratory workers and taxidermists.

○   **In what occupations are workers at risk of <u>organic mercury</u> exposure?**

Manufacturers of drugs/vaccines, fungicides, pesticides, wood preservatives, and farmers, and embalmers.

CADMIUM

○ **What is the chemical symbol for cadmium?**

Cd.

○ **What color is cadmium in its elemental state?**

Blue-white, lusterous metal or a grayish-white powder.

○ **Where is cadmium found in nature?**

Cadmium is a natural element in the earth's crust usually found as a cadmium oxide, cadmium chloride, cadmium sulfate, or cadmium sulfide.

○ **In nature, Cd is almost always found in conjunction with what element?**

Zinc.

○ **Which industrial processes and products may utilize cadmium?**

Fire detection systems, electrical cables and in some solders; in pigments for plastics, ceramics and glasses; in stabilizers for polyvinylchloride; as a protective plating on steel; nickel-cadmium battery manufacture, welding, electroplating.

○ **How may the general population potentially be exposed to cadmium?**

Breathing cigarette smoke, eating cadmium contaminated food.

○ **How much Cd is contained in cigarette smoke?**

16 micrograms of Cd per 20 cigarettes.

○ **What are the environmental (atmospheric) sources for cadmium?**

Cadmium enters air from mining, industry, and burning coal and household wastes.

○ **How does tap water becomes contaminated with Cd?**

Soft tap, water that lies in galavanized or black polyethylene pipe overnight may accumulate large amounts of Cd from the pipe material.

❍   **What is the EPA regulation regarding how much cadmium may be present in drinking water?**

5 parts per billion (ppb).

❍   **What is the FDA limit for cadmium in food colors?**

15 parts per million (ppm).

❍   **What are the clinical findings that may be consistent with the inhalation of cadmium containing fumes or dusts?**

Ocular and mucous membrane irritation, headache, dizziness, chills, fever, chest pain, metallic taste, headache, dyspnea, chest pains, cough with foamy or bloody sputum, and muscular weakness.

❍   **By what route is cadmium best absorbed?**

Inhalation

Cadmium is absorbed more efficiently by the lungs (30 to 60%) than by the gastrointestinal tract.

❍   **Which organs tend to accumulate cadmium?**

Liver, kidneys.

❍   **How is cadmium metabolized?**

There is essentially no direct metabolic conversions of cadmium. Rather, it binds to various proteins and macromolecules.

❍   **What is the principle route of excretion for cadmium?**

Urine.

❍   **What is the biological half-life of cadmium in the human body?**

17-30 years.

❍   **What is the most serious chronic effect of oral exposure to cadmium?**

Renal toxicity. Renal tubular proteinuria is the primary toxic effect of long-term cadmium exposure.

❍   **What condition has been associated with dietary intake of cadmium causing osteomalacia, osteoporosis and spontaneous fractures, originally documented in postmenopausal women in cadmium-contaminated areas of Japan?**

"Itai, itai" disease. *(Ouch- Ouch)*

❍   **What effect may chronic cadmium exposure have on the blood pressure?**

Hypertension.

❍   **What is the mechanism for the development of hypertension associated with cadmium exposure?**

This phenomenon is not currently well understood.

❍   **Does Cd cross the placenta?**

Yes.

❍   **Is cadmium a proven respiratory tract carcinogen?**

Inhalation exposure to cadmium may be associated with an increased incidence of respiratory tract cancer however epidemiologic evidence for this effect is very limited.

❍   **Is cadmium a human teratogen?**

Definitive data is not available regarding the developmental or reproductive toxicity of cadmium or cadmium compounds in humans.

❍   **How does IARC classify cadmium with regard to carcinogenic potential?**

IARC classifies cadmium and cadmium compounds as carcinogenic to humans (Group 1).

❍   **What effect does Acidification of cadmium-containing soils and sediments have on the concentration of cadmium in surface water and crops?**

Acidification of cadmium-containing soils and sediments may increase the concentrations of cadmium in surface waters and crops.

❍   **Does occupational exposure to cadmium cause prostate cancer?**

Several early studies reported an increased risk for prostate cancer in cadmium workers, but the results of later studies were not consistent.

❍   **Does occupational exposure to cadmium cause lung cancer?**

Early and recent studies provide consistent evidence that the risk for lung cancer is increased among workers exposed to cadmium.

❍   **What is the most likely mechanism for Cd toxicity?**

Cd noncompetitively inhibits calcium ion transport across the small intestine. It also reduces calcium ions absorption. It is the negative calcium balance that leads to the osteomalacia induced by Cd.

○   **What are the normal excretion characteristics for Cd?**

20% in urine.
70-80% in feces.

○   **What were the historical medicinal uses for Cd?**

Used in the treatment of syphilis, Tb and malaria.

○   **What are the most common clinical effects in chronic Cd poisoning?**

COPD, anosmia, dental yellowing, marked proteinuria.

○   **What were the clinical characteristics of "iai, itai" disease?**

Severe bone pain, waddling gait, aminoaciduria, glycosuria, decreased pancreatic function, marked osteomalacia, multiple pathological fractures.

○   **What percent of the original patients afflicted by itai itai disease died?**

50%.

○   **What is the specific treatment for acute and/or chronic Cd poisoning?**

There is no specific treatment.

SOLVENTS

○ **What are the main routes of exposure to aromatic solvents?**

Pulmonary and dermal.

○ **What combination of solvents is added to gasoline to elevate the octane rating?**

BTX (benzene, toluene and xylene).

○ **Which soil characteristic favors the evaporation of toluene when it is added to the soil: high organic content or low organic content?**

Toluene vaporizes more readily in hot, dry soil with little organic content.

○ **Which bacteria are responsible for soil degradation of toluene?**

Pseudomonas and Achroobacter.

○ **What is the main human urinary metabolite of toluene?**

Hippuric acid (75%).

○ **What are the clinical effects of acute toluene inhalation?**

Euphoria, headache, lightheadedness, ataxia, nausea, and sedation.

○ **What CNS lesion is associated with chronic inhalational toluene exposure?**

Diffuse demyelination.

○ **What are the clinical effects of chronic toluene inhalation?**

Ataxia, optic neuropathy, and tremor.

○ **What acid/base and electrolyte abnormalities are associated with chronic inhalation of toluene?**

Renal tubular acidosis, hypokalemia and hypophosphatemia.

○ **Is toluene carcinogenic?**

No.

❍ **What test is used to monitor workers who are exposed to toluene?**

Urine hippuric acid.

❍ **Are solvents found in cigarette smoke?**

Yes. Xylene and other solvents are found in cigarette smoke.

❍ **What are the possible clinical effects of chronic inhalational xylene?**

Headache, fatigue and memory deficits.

❍ **What test is used for biological monitoring of xylene exposure?**

Urine methylhippuric acids.

❍ **What enzymes are necessary to metabolize xylene to methylhippuric acids?**

P450 enzymes, alcohol dehydrogenase, and aldehyde dehydrogenase.

❍ **What work-related factor increases the absorption of styrene, toluene, and xylene in workers?**

Physical exercise.

❍ **What is considered the "toxic" metabolite of styrene?**

7,8-styrene oxide.

❍ **What co-inhalants can alter the metabolism of styrene?**

(TCE)
Trichloroethylene and toluene decrease styrene metabolism.

❍ **What are the clinical effects of an acute inhalation exposure to styrene?**

Mucous membrane irritation, headache, nausea, lightheadedness and confusion.

❍ **What peripheral nerve effects have been associated with exposure to styrene?**

Longer latency on peripheral nerve conduction studies.

❍ **What test is used as a biological monitor for exposure to styrene?**

Urine mendelic acid.

❍ **Does ethanol use have any effect on styrene metabolism?**

Yes. Chronic ethanol use can induce the P450 enzymes and increase the metabolism of styrene to 7,8-styrene.

○ **What CNS effects have been associated with chronic exposure to styrene?**

Ataxia, alterations in hearing and vision, and EEG changes.

○ **What is the proposed mechanism of 7,8-styrene neurotoxicity?**

Alkylation of DNA.

○ **What effect does dimethylformamide have on alcohol dehydrogenase?**

Dimethylformamide inhibits alcohol dehydrogenase.

○ **What reaction occurs when workers who use dimethylformamide ingest ethanol?**

A disulfiram-like reaction with flushing, vomiting, chest tightness and dyspnea.

○ **What hepatic effect is associated with a large acute exposure to dimethylformamide?**

Centrilobular necrosis.

○ **What are the two forms of naphtha?**

Petroleum distillate naphtha and coal tar naphtha.

○ **What is the Stoddard solvent?**

A mixture of hydrocarbons with carbon chains ranging from C7 through C12.

○ **What are white spirits?**

A mixture of hydrocarbons with carbon chains ranging from C7 through C11.

○ **What are the clinical effects of an acute inhalational exposure to a high concentration of Stoddard solvent?**

Headache, vomiting, coma, mucosal irritation and pneumonitis.

○ **What are the dermatological effects of Stoddard solvent?**

Dermatitis with erythema, vesicles, ulceration, desquamation and crusting.

○ **Is Stoddard solvent considered carcinogenic?**

No.

○ **What is the primary metabolite of isopropanol?**

Acetone.

○ **What are the clinical effects of acute isopropanol ingestion?**

Euphoria, sedation, vomiting, diarrhea and hypotension.

○ **What enzyme metabolizes methanol?**

Alcohol dehydrogenase.

○ **What methanol metabolite produces a metabolic acidosis?**

Formate (formic acid).

○ **What methanol metabolite is responsible for the ocular effects of methanol toxicity?**

Formate (formic acid).

○ **What can be used to decrease the metabolism from methanol to formate?**

4-methylpyrazole or ethanol.

○ **What are the clinical effects of chronic exposure to methyl-ethyl-ketone (MEK) at 90 ppm?**

None.

○ **What are the clinical effects of dermal exposure to dimethyl ester?**

Delayed-onset caustic burns.

○ **What are the clinical effects of acute inhalational exposure to dimethyl ester?**

Coma, pulmonary edema, renal and hepatic failure, seizures and death.

○ **What are the clinical effects of chronic exposure to tri-ortho-cresyl phosphate?**

Motor neuropathy.

○ **What pulmonary disorder is associated with exposure to chloromethyl ethers?**

Pulmonary cancer, specifically small-cell cancer.

○ **What are the clinical effects of exposure to glycidyl ethers?**

Mucosal irritation and dermal burns.

○ **What metabolite of ethylene glycol causes a metabolic acidosis?**

Glycolic acid.

○ **What metabolite of ethylene glycol may form crystals in the urine?**

Oxalate (oxalic acid) forms calcium oxalate crystals.

○ **What are the clinical effects of acute ingestion of ethylene glycol?**

Euphoria followed by acidosis, hypotension and renal failure.

○ **What test is used as a biological monitor of styrene exposure?**

Urine mandelic acid.

○ **What are the clinical effects of acute exposure to dioxane?**

Mucous membrane irritation, sedation, headache, vomitting, pulmonary edema, renal and hepatic damage.

○ **What enzyme metabolizes ethylene glycol?**

Alcohol dehydrogenase.

CHEMICAL CARCINOGENESIS

(Initiation)

✳ O T/F: Cancer is a multistep process that includes ~~induction~~, promotion, and progression.

True.

O The prevention of environmental and occupational cancers can best be accomplished by elimination of what product?

Tobacco.

O The prevention of environmental and occupational cancers can best be accomplished by the use of what agent?

Sun blocking agent.

O T/F: Cancer is the second leading cause of death in the United States. *(Heart Dz. #1)*

True.

O T/F: Benign tumors can be derived from abnormally growing tissues.

False. Benign tumors can be derived from normally growing tissues.

✳ O Malignant tumors are derived from either the epidermis (ectoderm and endoderm) or the _____.

Mesenchyma.

✳ O Epithelially derived malignant tumors are termed_____.

Carcinomas.

O Malignant tumors of mesenchymal origin are called ____.

Sarcomas.

O T/F: A slow growth pattern predominates for benign tumors and more rapidly dividing pattern for malignant tumors.

True.

○ **T/F: Chemical carcinogenesis category ratings of 1 or A signify ample evidence to include the chemical as a carcinogen in humans.**

True.

○ **What are the three essential steps to Carcinogenesis?**

Initiation, Promotion, Progression.

○ **What can cause genetic damage from either a single base pair substitution or a gross chromosomal change?**

Chemicals.

○ **What normal cellular genes, when <u>activated</u>, inappropriately as oncogenes, cause altered regulation of growth and differentiation pathways?**

Protooncogenes.

○ **What normal cellular genes, when <u>inactivated,</u> may cause dysregulation of growth and differentiation pathway, enhancing the probability of neoplastic transformation?**

Tumor suppression genes.

○ **In colon cancer, three tumor suppressor genes and one protooncogene are frequently altered. What are they?**

MCC, p53, DCC, and K-ras.

○ **T/F: It is commonly held that each tumor is descended from a single altered cell, referred to as a monoclonal in origin.**

True.

○ **What can an electrophilic chemical that can covalently bind to the cell's DNA do?**

Attack a cell.

○ **Name 4 genetic changes induced by chemical carcinogens.**

Gene mutation, gene amplifications, chromosomal rearrangement and aneuploidy.

○ **The initial interaction of a chemical with DNA is known as what?**

Initiation.

○   **What do tumor promoters facilitate?**

Clonal expansion.

○   **T/F: Progression is the process that allows the cells to become malignant cancers.**

True.

○   **T/F: Initiators are not carcinogenic in and of themselves and do not bind to DNA.**

False. Promoters are not carcinogenic and do not bind to DNA.

○   **What two ways can carcinogens be categorized?**

Primary or procarcinogens.

○   **Primary carcinogens directly act with _____ as a genotoxin.**

DNA.

○   **T/F: Procarcinogens require metabolic activation before it can interact with the genome.**

True.

○   **Most xenobiotics associated with the development of cancer require some type of metabolic alteration. What conversion does this typically involve?**

Conversion to highly reactive electrophils.

○   **Methylene chloride is oxidized by _____ in various rodent models.**

P450 IIE1.

○   **Name several mechanisms by which protooncogenes may alter growth or differentiation.**

Point mutation, chromosome translocation or gene amplification.

○   **T/F: Chemical carcinogens that require metabolic activation are called "direct acting" chemical carcinogens.**

False, they are called "indirect acting".

○   **Precarcinogens or procarcinogens are other ways to describe what type of carcinogens?**

Indirect acting.

O   **By what method may indirect acting xenobiotics, including carcinogens, be detoxified?**

By oxidation.

O   **Detoxification by oxidation reactions occur via what system?**

P450 system.

(Primary Carcinogens)

O   **T/F: Direct acting carcinogens are by their nature chemically unstable.**

True.

O   **Give some examples of direct acting carcinogens.**

Ethyleneimine, b-propiolactone, bis (chloromethyl) ether, bis (chloromethyl) ether, bis (2-chlorol-ethyl) sulfide, diepoxybutane.

O   **Many of the above mentioned direct acting carcinogen compounds act as alkylators of what?**

Cellular macromolecules.

O   **Genotoxic carcinogens are those chemicals that react directly with what material?**

Genetic material.

O   **T/F: Only direct acting carcinogens may function as genotoxic carcinogens.**

False, both direct and indirect acting carcinogens may function as genotoxic carcinogens.

O   **Non-genotoxic or epigenetic carcinogens do not bind to DNA but may form what?**

Adducts with other cellular constituents.

O   **T/F: It is not known whether carcinogens act as initiators by causing point mutations activating oncogenes, by causing deletions in growth suppressors genes or by acting on elements that regulate transcription or induce changes in DNA amplification.**

True.

O   **Name two materials that may act as epigenetic carcinogens.**

Films and fibers.

❍ **Give examples of certain physiochemical factors that may lead to the development of cancer by epigenetic mechanisms.**

Osmolarity, Ph.

❍ **What is the term used to describe specific chemicals capable of causing specific tumors in specific organs?**

Organotropism.

❍ **Name a chemical that is known to induce angiosarcomas of the liver in rats, mice, hamsters, as well as humans.**

Vinyl chloride.

❍ **How are transgenic cells created?**

When a specific gene is introduced, along with a promoter, into a cell to determine tumor induction upon exposure to a specific chemical or substrate.

❍ **T/F: Transgenic mice have been shown to respond within just weeks to months when exposed to a carcinogen.**

True.

❍ **T/F: Experimental animals have been created that have had certain genes deleted or "knocked out."**

True.

❍ **T/F: Researchers have created pairs of mice that differ by a factor of 100 in their risk for tumor development.**

True.

❍ **An important growth inhibitory protein has recently been identified which may play a role in the suppression of premalignant cell changes. What is it?**

Transforming growth factor-β (TGF-β).

❍ **A common biological marker, called _____ is a serum test that is used in the diagnosis and screening of prostate cancer.**

PSA (prostate specific antigen).

O   **What is the name of a common biological marker, a protein that is used to monitor patients during treatment for colon and breast cancer?**

CEA (carcinoembryonic antigen).

O   **Name some serum biomarkers used to assist in the diagnosis of carcinomas of the testes, liver and pancreas, respectively?**

Alpha-fetoprotein (α-FP), beta-human choriogonadotropin hormone (β-HCG), and CA19-9.

O   **T/F: The BRCA1 is a genetic biomarker which was first identified in 1990 by Hall, et al at the University of California in Berkeley.**

True.

O   **T/F: Women who are heterozygous for mutations, which involve the truncation of the protein, of BRCA1 and BRCA1 genes have up to a 90% lifetime risk for cancer of the breast, colon, ovary, and other sites with an early age of onset.**

True.

O   **A cluster is an aggregation, real or perceived of some particular adverse health event grouped by what two things?**

Time and space.

O   **T/F: To demonstrate a clustering of cancers, they must, de facto, be identical.**

True.

O   **During the investigation of a cancer cluster what two things should be reviewed for accuracy of diagnosis?**

Histopathology and medical records.

O   **T/F: Latency of time to occurrence is an important identifier in cancer cluster cases.**

True.

O   **When comparing observed number of cases to expected number of cases, the expected number can be obtained from what resource?**

Cancer registries.

○ **Define latency period.**

Period of time from onset of exposure to a chemical or environment to the appearance of clinically identifiable disease. *(symptoms)*

○ **What is the estimated latency period for solid tumors?**

15-20 years.

○ **What is the estimated latency period for hematologic tumors?**

5-10 years.

○ **Smoking is considered a confounding and/or contributing factor in implicating a chemical or environment. Name some others.**

Substance abuse, genetic history, other potential exposures, type of employment and hobbies.

○ **T/F: A true "cluster" is unlikely if there is a mixture of cancer types.**

True.

○ **Asbestos has been associated with what cancer?**

Lung.

○ **Arsenic has been associated with what cancers?** *(Inorganic)*

Lung, skin., *bladder, Liver*

○ **What cancer type is associated with large exposures to benzene?**

Acute myelogenous leukemia. *(AML)*

○ **Wood dust has shown an association with what type of cancer?**

Nasal.

○ **Commercial fishing may be associated with what type of cancer?** *(lots of sun exposure)*

Skin. *(Dermal)*

○ **Tobacco smoke is categorized by IARC as what?**

Known human carcinogen "1."

○ **Large exposures to <u>vinyl chloride</u> has been associated with what type of cancer?**

Angiosarcoma of the liver.

○ **What is a carcinogen?**

A substance of process that is capable of causing an increased number of tumors in test species.

○ **What is a procarcinogen?**

A substance that becomes a carcinogen after being metabolic activated.

○ **T/F: Most cancers display some chromosomal abnormalities.**

True.

○ **Cancer <u>promotion is</u> characterized by?**

Reversibility, morphologic changes, noninitiation, modulation and threshold.

○ **T/F: Defective DNA repair predisposes to cancer.**

True.

→ Testicular/Skin / ? Lung

○ **<u>Ionizing radiation</u> has been most commonly associated with what cancers?**

Breast and thyroid.

↖ Radioactive Iodine

WORKPLACE DRUG TESTING

○ **Substance abuse is estimated to cost the United States how much annually?**

$200 Billion.

○ **Are certain job categories more prone to substance abuse?**

Yes.

○ **What job categories are more prone to substance abuse?**

Construction workers.

○ **In 1988, what were the percentage positives in construction workers?**

17%.

○ **What job categories are least prone to substance abuse?**

Teachers, police officers and child care workers.

○ **What is the estimate of adults who abuse alcohol and drugs?**

10-40%.

○ **What is the estimated number of workers who are substance abusers?**

30 million.

○ **Have drug testing programs led to a decrease in substance abuse?**

Yes.

○ **What federal agency has promulgated drug testing regulations?**

Department of transpiration. _transportation_ _(DOT)_

○ **What agency oversees the pipeline industry?**

RSPA - Research and Special Projects Administration.

○ **How many drugs were allowed to be tested for in the original DOT mandate?**

5 drugs (marijuana, cocaine, amphetamines, opiates and phencyclidine).

○ **In what year was the Drug Free Work Place Act enacted?**

1988.

○ **In 1990 the DOT testing program was extended to include which group?**

Small trucking companies.

○ **What is the volume of urine required for split specimen collection?**

45-ml.

○ **If a donor is unable to provide a urine sample, DOT testing calls for drinking what volume of fluids?**

40 ounces over a 3-hour time period.

○ **What was the percentage of positive urines in 1988?**

13%.

○ **What was the percentage of positive urines in 1998?**

6%.

○ **Prior to breath testing for alcohol, what was the percentage of construction workers reporting heavy use of ethanol?**

21%.

○ **Are workers who test positive for drugs or alcohol more prone to involuntary turnover?**

Yes.

○ **Employees that tested positive for illegal drugs, what was their absenteeism rate?**

59.3 % higher than those testing negative.

○ **In one US Postal Service study, donors testing positive of marijuana was predicative of?**

Increased turnover, accidents, injuries, disciplinary actions and absenteeism.

○ **According to 49 CFR 382.305, how must randomization be done?**

Scientifically valid method (random number table, computer generated random number list).

○ **Random drug testing is most effective in detecting what?**

Frequent users of illicit drugs.

○ **One study found that 50% of random positives are from?**

Everyday users.

○ **In the same study, what percentage of positives was from infrequent users?**

7%.

○ **In 1996, what was the percentage of positives for pre-employment tests?**

4.3%.

○ **In 1996, what was the percentage of positives for random tests?**

2.9%.

○ **In 1996, what was the percentage of positives for post-accident tests?**

3.3%.

○ **In 1996, what was the percentage of positives in for-cause testing?**

11%.

○ **In 1996, what was the percentage of positives for return to duty tests?**

3.8%.

○ **Excluding alcohol, what substance is most likely to be found in tests?**

Marijuana.

○ **Excluding alcohol, what substance is least likely to be found in tests?**

Phencyclidine. *(PCP)*

○ **What is NIDA?**

National Institute of Drug Abuse.

○ **What is SAMHSA?**

Substance Abuse and Mental Health Services Administration.

○ **What are the NIDA-5 drugs?**

Marijuana, cocaine, amphetamine, opiates and phencyclidine.

○ **What is the media preferred for testing, excluding alcohol?**

Urine.

○ **What media is preferred for alcohol testing?**

Breath.

○ **In non-DOT testing, how often are benzodiazepines detected?**

0.38%.

○ **How is a donor identified?**

Picture identification.

○ **How is a donor identified, if they have no picture ID?**

Employer representative.

○ **If there is no ID or employer representative, how is the donor identified?**

Two forms of non-picture ID bearing the donor's signature.

○ **What is the required temperature range for recently collected urine?**

90–100 degrees F.

○ **A sample with a temperature less than 90 degrees is suggestive of?**

Tampering by dilution or substitution.

○ **The tamper-resistant seal is placed on the collection container by the collector. What is the next step?**

The seal is initialed and dated by the collector, and initialed by the donor.

○ **If a donor appears intoxicated, the collector may?**

Collect a sample under direct observation.

○ **A split-collection is divided in the presence of?**

The donor.

○ **What is the required volume in split-sample collection for specimen A?**

30 ml.

○ **What is the required volume in split-sample collection for specimen B?**

15 ml.

○ **In DOT split-specimen testing, both bottles are sent to?**

The initial laboratory.

○ **In DOT split-specimen testing, if bottle A test positive, how long is bottle A retained?**

Minimum of 1 year.

○ **In DOT split-specimen testing, if bottle A test positive, how long is bottle B retained?**

At least 60 days.

○ **In split-specimen testing, if bottle A tests positive for one drug, what can bottle B be analyzed for?**

Only for the positive analyte in bottle A.

○ **Bottle B is tested at what detection limits?**

LOD - limits of detection.

○ **Are overnight carriers appropriate for sample transportation to laboratories?**

Yes.

○ **How many parts does the custody and control form have?**

Seven.

○ **Who must sign the custody and control form?**

Anyone handling the specimen.

○ **Can laboratories test for adulterants?**

Yes.

○ **What are typical tests for adulteration?**

Creatinine, specific gravity, pH, nitrite concentration.

○ **Screening tests are typically done by what method?**

Immunoassay.

○ **What is the most common confirmation methodology?**

Gas chromatograph coupled with mass spectroscopy (GC/MS).

○ **IF a screening test is positive, DOT guidelines suggest what method for confirmation?**

GC/MS.

○ **What are the screening/confirmation cutoff levels for amphetamines?**

1000 ng/ml and 500 ng/ml.

○ **What are the screening/confirmation cutoff levels for phencyclidine?**

25 ng/ml and 25 ng/ml.

○ **What is the target analyte for marijuana?**

Delta-9-THC-acid.

○ **What are the screening/confirmation cutoff levels for marijuana?**

50 ng/ml and 15 ng/ml.

○ **What is the target analyte for cocaine?**

Benzoylecgonine.

○ **How long may urine samples be positive in marijuana users?**

1 day to 3 weeks.

○ **What is an MRO?**

Medical review officer, physician determining validity of test result.

○ **With a laboratory positive test, the MRO contacts the donor to determine if there is a?**

Alternative medical explanation for the positive test.

○ **Is there a legitimate indication for a urine positive for phencyclidine?**

No.

○ **Are MRO's mandated in a formal role in alcohol breath testing?**

No.

○ **In DOT testing, a donor with a confirmed positive must be referred to?**

Certified employee assistance program.

○ **What common drug are codeine and heroin metabolized to?**

Morphine.

○ **What is the intermediate metabolism of heroin to morphine?**

6-monoacetyl morphine (6-MAM).

○ **The presence of 6-MAM is indicative of?**

Heroin use.

ERGONOMICS

○ **What are the goals of ergonomics in the workplace?**

Increase productivity.
Reduce risk of work-related musculoskeletal disorders (WMSD's).
Increase safety and quality of work by decreasing fatigue and errors.

○ **List 7 ergonomic risk factors**

Vibration – segmental or whole-body.
Force.
Position – awkward postures, static postures.
Repetition.
Duration.
Compression.
Temperature – heat injury, Raynaud's phenomenon.
(Memory tool mnemonic: "Very Few People Really Develop Carpal Tunnel").

○ **If an ergonomist knows the work intensity of a task, (s)he can make recommendations to modify the task or modify the performance of the task. What objective measures can be used to estimate work intensity?**

Respiratory rate.
Cardiac output (heart rate).
Metabolic rate – calorimetry, oxygen uptake.
Core body temperature.

○ **T/F: Work-rest scheduling is one method to ensure workers do not exceed their physical work capacity.**

True.

○ **The neutral posture of a joint is determined by the _____ (minimum, maximum, resting) length of the muscle crossing that joint.**

Resting.

○ **The muscle in which position is capable of generating the greatest force: muscle extended, muscle at resting length, muscle contracted?**

Muscle at resting length.

❍   **To maintain neutral posture, objects that are being lifted or worked on should be kept close to the body and in the _____ zone.**

Strike.

❍   **Regarding biomechanics, the components that comprise a moment are _____ and _____.**

Force – the weight of an object.
Distance from the body – perpendicular distance from the axis of rotation.

❍   **Regarding biomechanics, 3 classes of levers can be described using the relationship between the force, resistance, and fulcrum. Describe the 3 classes of levers.**

First class lever – the fulcrum is between the force and the resistance.
Second class lever – the resistance is between the force and the fulcrum.
Third class lever – the force is between the resistance and the fulcrum.

❍   **Regarding biomechanics and levers, in which circumstance is mechanical advantage present?**

When the force arm is longer than the resistance arm. Force arm is the distance between the fulcrum and the force. Resistance arm is the distance between the fulcrum and the resistance.

❍   **Third class levers never have mechanical advantage, so they are adapted for speed and range of motion rather than _____.**

Strength.

❍   **When applying anthropometric design principles and designing for the extreme, clearance requirements (doorways, manholes, etc.) are determined by the _____ (largest or smallest) worker; reach requirements are determined by the _____ (largest or smallest) worker.**

Largest.
Smallest.

❍   **Regarding anthropometric design, most human body dimensions are normally distributed; therefore __ tables are used to determine the range of body dimensions for given percentiles.**

Z.

❍   **Approximately how many pounds of force are required to strike a key on a keyboard?**

1 pound.

O   **In general, what range of distance should a computer monitor be from the operator's eyes?**

18-30 inches.

O   **Regarding office ergonomics, the top of the computer monitor should generally be: at eye level, 2 inches below eye level, or 2 inches above eye level?**

At eye level.

O   **Regarding office ergonomics, is the most appropriate use of keyboard wrist rests is for constant contact while typing or for intermittent resting between typing tasks?**

Keyboard wrist rests are for resting, not "parking."

O   **Regarding office ergonomics, an articulating keyboard platform should be adjustable in which dimensions?**

Forward and backward.
Up and down.
Pitch.

O   **The traditional telephone handset can be associated with awkward postures and compression in the neck and shoulder region. If appropriate and feasible, 2 replacement options include _____ or _____.**

Headset.
Speakerphone.

O   **If an office worker's chair is adjusted so high that his/her feet do not touch the floor, a _____ effectively raises the level of the floor to relieve pressure on the popliteal region behind the knees.**

Footrest.

O   **To avoid eye strain due to _____, a computer monitor should never be placed directly in front of a window.**

Direct glare.

O   **The NIOSH recommended lifting limit is __ pounds under optimal conditions.**

51.

❍   **List the 5 categories of manual material handling (a 6th category would be a combination of these 5).**

Lifting.
Lowering.
Carrying.
Pulling.
Pushing.

❍   **Powered handtools are faster, stronger, and more efficient than handtools, but the tradeoff for this increased speed and power is an increased exposure to _____.**

Vibration.

❍   **What term describes brightness within the field of vision that causes discomfort, eye fatigue, or interference with vision?**

Glare.

❍   **List the 4 methods of heat exchange.**

Conduction.
Convection.
Radiation.
Evaporation.

❍   **What are the 6 variables used to compute the Strain Index for ergonomic job analysis?**

Intensity of exertion.
Duration of Exertion.
Exertions per minute.
Hand/wrist posture.
Speed of work.
Duration of task (per day).

❍   **The NIOSH lifting equation considers 6 task variables when determining the recommended weight limit for a task or job. What are these 6 variables?**

Horizontal distance.
Vertical distance.
Travel distance.
Couplings (handles).
Frequency of lift.
Duration of lift.

❍ **When job requirements exceed biomechanical capability, the worker is at risk for an overexertion injury. Which physiologic model for assessing job requirements compares the aerobic demand of a job to consensus levels of acceptable aerobic demands?**

Energy expenditure model.

❍ **What term describes the transient loss of work capacity resulting from preceding work?**

Fatigue.

❍ **To prevent the symptoms of Carpal Tunnel Syndrome, wrist braces are frequently recommended for use at night. How does this treatment minimize symptoms?**

When sleeping, the wrist can assume an extreme posture, increasing the carpal tunnel pressure. The braces maintain the wrist(s) in a neutral posture, keeping the carpal tunnel pressure below the ischemic threshold.

❍ **What is the study of the mechanical interaction between workers and their work environment for the purpose of modifying workplace design to maximize worker efficiency and worker health.**

Ergonomics.

❍ **What is another name for ergonomics?**

Human Factors Engineering.

❍ **Regarding ergonomic hazards, list the sources of physical stressors.**

Excessive job demands.
Improperly designed workstations, tools, or equipment.
Inappropriate work techniques.
Excessive work rates.
Machine-paced work vs. self-paced work.
Inadequate rest-to-work ratio.
Restriction of worker body movement.

CARPAL TUNNEL SYNDROME

О **What is the prevalence of symptomatic carpal tunnel syndrome?**

3% among women, 2% among men.

О **What is the peak prevalence age for carpal tunnel syndrome in women?**

55 years of age.

О **Where is the carpal tunnel located?**

The carpal tunnel is located at the base of the palm just distal to the distal wrist crease.

О **Where is the boundaries of the carpal tunnel?**

The carpal tunnel is bounded on three sides by the carpal bones, which create an arch and on the palmar side by the fibrous flexor retinaculum or transverse carpal ligament.

О **What is the cause for carpal tunnel syndrome?**

Carpal tunnel syndrome is caused by elevated pressure in the carpal tunnel causing ischemia of the median nerve.

О **What may happen as a result of prolonged or frequent episodes of elevated pressure in the carpal tunnel?**

Segmental demyelination and increasing symptoms.

О **What are occurs with prolonged ischemia within the carpal tunnel?**

Axonal injury and potentially reversible nerve dysfunction.

О **What are the medical conditions that may be associated with carpal tunnel syndrome?**

Pregnancy, fracture, amyloidosis, hypothyroidism, diabetes, acromegaly, steroid use and the use of estrogens.

О **What percentage of case of carpal tunnel syndrome occur in association with the above listed medical problems?**

Up to 30% of case of carpal tunnel syndrome occur in association with these medical conditions.

❍   **What percentage of patient's with carpal tunnel syndrome have diabetes mellitus?**

Approximately 6%.

❍   **What specific activities are associated with the development of carpal tunnel syndrome?**

Repetitive activities of the hand and wrist, especially those that combine force and repetitive activity.

❍   **What occupations are associated with the high incidence of carpal tunnel syndrome?**

Food processing, manufacturing, logging, and construction work.

❍   **What is the natural history of carpal tunnel syndrome?**

The nerve conduction abnormalities tend to worsen overtime.

❍   **How is carpal tunnel syndrome diagnosed?**

Carpal tunnel syndrome is diagnosed using a combination of electrodiagnostic studies as well as symptom complex.

❍   **Symptoms consistent with carpal tunnel syndrome occur in approximately what percentage of the population _____?**

15%.

❍   **Carpal tunnel syndrome produces what sets of symptoms?**

Pain, tingling, numbness, or combination of these symptoms.

❍   **Loss of two-point discrimination in a median nerve distribution as well as thenar atrophy occur in carpal tunnel syndrome at what stage of its pathophysiology?**

These are late findings.

❍   **What provocative test may assist in the diagnosis of carpal tunnel syndrome?**

Phalen's maneuver and Tinel's sign.

❍   **What is Phalen's maneuver?**

Phalen's maneuver is having the patient report if flexion of the wrist for one minute produces pain or paresthesias in the distribution of the median nerve.

❍ **What is Tinel's sign?**

Tinel's sign is judged to be present if tapping lightly over the volar surface of the wrist causes radiating paresthesias in the digits innervated by the median nerve.

❍ **What is the treatment for carpal tunnel syndrome.**

Treatment for carpal tunnel syndrome includes a combination of splinting, medications, local fluid, steroid injections and surgery.

❍ **What percentage of patients will have these symptoms of carpal tunnel syndrome symptom relieved with using of wrist splint.**

80%.

❍ **Injections of steroids can improve symptoms in what percentage of patient's with carpal tunnel syndrome?**

75%.

❍ **What is the surgical approach to the treatment of carpal tunnel syndrome?**

Carpal tunnel release surgery is the approach.

❍ **What alternative therapies for carpal tunnel syndrome has been attempted?**

Acupuncture, chiropractic manipulation and yoga, none of which have proven to be effective.

NOISE

- ○ **What bone is attached to the eardrum?**

Malleus.

- ○ **To what membrane does the stapes attach?**

Oval window.

- ○ **Vibrations of the oval window are transmitted into the?**

Fluid-filled scala vestibuli.

- ○ **Where is the oval window located?**

Between the vestibular apparatus and the cochlea.

- ○ **What is a Hertz?**

Cycles per second.

- ○ **What is the range of frequencies that may be appreciated by the human ear?**

20 to 20,000 Hz.

- ○ **How is sound transmitted through air?**

In waveform compressions of the air adjacent to a vibrating surface.

- ○ **How is sound different than noise?**

Noise is unwanted sound.

- ○ **What are the numbers of pressure peaks passed in 1 second?**

The frequency measure din Hertz.

- ○ **The subjective perception of a tone is called?**

Pitch.

- ○ **What two factors are important in assessing adverse effects of noise?**

Frequency spectrum and intensity.

○   **Sound intensity is measured in what units?**

Decibels (dB).

○   **What are decibels?**

Sound pressure levels (Lp) measured in a log scale.

○   **A dB represents what percent of a Bel?**

10 percent.

○   **What are two methods for assessing noise?**

Frequency analysis and loudness levels.

○   **What is used to measure frequency analysis?**

An octave band analyzer.

○   **What units are used to measure loudness?**

Phons.

○   **What is a Phon?**

Numerically the same as dB values of an equally loud 1000 Hz sound.

○   **What are five potential health issues related to noise?**

Annoyance, interference with speech and phone conversations, and hearing loss.

○   **What is the noise level found in normal conversation?**

50 dB

○   **What is the noise level associated with thunder?**

120 dB

○   **What is the noise level associated with using a chain saw?**

110 dB

❍   **What is the noise level 50 feet from a typical diesel truck?**

40 dB

❍   **What is the noise level of shouted conversation?**

90 dB

❍   **What is the noise level during cotton spinning?**

83 dB

❍   **What is the noise level of a riveting machine?**

110 dB

❍   **What is the noise level 100 feet from a rock drill?**

92 dB

❍   **What is the sound associated with an after-burner of a jet aircraft?**

150 dB

❍   **What process presents the greatest risk for hearing loss?**

Military operations.

❍   **What is the OSHA PEL-TWA for noise?**

90 dB

❍   **What is the ACGIH TLV-TWA for noise?**

85 dB

❍   **When did OSHA first issue its Standard to prevent hearing loss?**

1983.

❍   **At what noise level does OSHA require employers to support a hearing conservation program?**

85 dB

O   **What are the most common symptom and sign of acute acoustic trauma?**

Hearing loss and tinnitus.

O   **With acute acoustic trauma, what frequency range is most affected?**

4,000 to 8,000 Hz.

O   **How long can it take to stabilize hearing loss in acute acoustical trauma?**

Weeks to months.

O   **What symptom most often prompts workers to seek medical attention after suffering acute acoustical trauma?**

Tinnitus.

O   **After a terrorist explosion in Northern Ireland, what percent of those present in the restaurant were found to have hearing loss one year later?**

30%.

O   **After acute acoustic trauma, what is the most common finding on examination?**

Normal examination.

O   **Beside audiometry, what test is useful in evaluating blast related hearing loss?**

Brain Stem Auditory Evoked Response (BAER).

O   **What are three complications following blast injury?**

Persistent perforation of TM, permanent hearing loss and cholesteatoma.

O   **Patients with persistent perforation should be advised to?**

Keep water and foreign bodies out of the meatus.

O   **After acute acoustic trauma, the German military has had some success with what medication?**

Dextran.

O   **Prolonged exposure to elevated noise principally damages?**

Inner ear.

○ **What cells of the inner ear are injured from chronic noise exposure?**

Organ of Corti.

○ **What other structures can be injured?**

The cochlear blood vessels, stria vascularis and nerve endings.

○ **What is the chronic hearing loss associated with aging termed?**

Presbycusis.

○ **If the oval window becomes ossified, as it can in otosclerosis. How is sound transmitted to the organ of Corti?**

Via vibrations transmitted through bone.

○ **Noise induced hearing loss generally tends to increase with aging, as well as?**

Duration of employment.

○ **What employment interval does most noise induced hearing loss tends to occur?**

First 10 years.

○ **Early noise induced hearing loss tends to affect?**

Higher-pitched consonant sounds.

○ **With noise induced hearing loss, speech is recognized less clearly as opposed to?**

Lower in volume.

○ **The major risk factor for noise induced hearing loss is?**

Prolonged unprotected exposure to noise in excess of 85 dB.

○ **A common cause of conduction deafness is?**

Cerumen accumulation.

○ **Deafness may be divided into how many categories?**

Five.

❍ **Interference of sound transmission to the inner ear is called?**

Conduction hearing loss.

❍ **Damage to the cochlear mechanism or auditory nerve is termed?**

Nerve deafness.

❍ **What is central deafness?**

Injury to sites in the brain.

❍ **What is diplacusis?**

False sense of pitch.

❍ **Epidemiological studies indicate that cigarette smokers have how much of a greater risk of noise induced hearing loss?**

40 per cent greater than non-smokers.

❍ **What solvent of abuse has been associated with haring impairment and balance disorders?**

Toluene.

❍ **Which hormonal levels are increased in response to noise?**

Urinary catecholamines and 17-hydroxycorticoids.

❍ **What common medical condition has shown a relationship with noise induced hearing loss?**

Hypertension.

❍ **As noise induced hearing loss progresses, the workers ability to appreciate what sounds are altered first?**

Soft sounds.

❍ **What sounds may be difficult to appreciate by a worker with noise induced hearing loss?**

High-pitched sounds.

❍ **How often is vertigo associated with noise induced hearing loss?**

Rarely.

○   **Vertigo may be a symptom of what condition?**

Acoustic neuroma.

○   **What major drugs are associated with deafness?**

Furosemide, aminoglycosides, analgesics and tricyclic antidepressants.

○   **What is a common cause of reversible medication induced tinnitus?**

Salicylates.

○   **In assessing noise induced hearing loss, thresholds above what level are considered abnormal?**

25 dB

○   **Early impairment of noise induced hearing loss tends to occur at what frequency?**

4,000 Hz.

○   **Workplace noise may be measured by either?**

Area or personal dosimetry.

○   **What is the preferred method to reduce noise in work settings?**

Engineering controls.

○   **How much attenuation does hearing-protection provide?**

15-30 dB.

○   **When earplugs are combined with earmuffs, show much addition attenuation can be achieved?**

An additional 10-15 dB.

VIBRATION

○ Occupational exposure to vibration trauma is a frequent cause of _____ , also known as "vibration white finger."

Raynaud's Phenomenon.

○ What is the largest population of vibration-exposed workers?

Commercial vehicle drivers.

○ What is the name of the clinical rating scheme, introduced in 1987, that established separate grading criteria for vascular and neurologic signs and symptoms in hand-arm vibration syndrome (HAVS)?

The Stockholm Scale.

○ The energy content of mechanical oscillation (vibration) is expressed in terms of _____.

Acceleration.

○ Regarding acceleration, 1 g = ___ m/sec².

9.8.

○ The time component of tool acceleration is referred to as the _____.

Root Mean Square (RMS).

○ Regarding vibration, what term describes the number of oscillations per second.

Frequency.

○ What is the unit of frequency?

Hertz (Hz).

○ What is the best method for evaluating injury to myelinated nerve fibers?

Nerve conduction studies.

○ Subjective discomfort is more dominant at (higher/lower) vibration frequencies.

Lower.

○   **What are the most damaging vibratory frequencies for nociceptive and vascular injury?**

200-500 Hz.

○   **Antivibration materials (gloves, tool wraps, etc.) are more effective at filtering out (higher/lower) frequency vibrations.**

Higher.

○   **What is the resonant frequency for whole-body vibration when sitting?**

5 Hz.

○   **What are the two broad categories of vibration exposure in humans?**

Whole-body vibration.
Segmental vibration (hand-arm vibration).

○   **Health effect from exposure to whole-body vibration generally occur as a result of what range of frequencies?**

1 – 100 Hz.

○   **What is the predominant health effect resulting from exposure to segmental vibration?**

Hand Arm Vibration Syndrome (HAVS).

○   **List the 3 components of Hand Arm Vibration Syndrome (HAVS).**

Circulatory disturbances (vasospasm, white finger).
Sensory/motor disturbances (numbness, loss of dexterity).
Musculoskeletal disturbances (muscle, bone, joint disorders).

○   **What is the best quantitative test for evaluating the vascular component of Hand Arm Vibration syndrome (HAVS)?**

Cold-challenge plethysmography.

○   **What term describes the periodic motion of a body in alternately opposite directions from a position of rest?**

Vibration.

❍   **What anatomic structure is the reference point for measurements of whole-body vibration (WBV)?**

Sternum.

❍   **According the internationally accepted coordinate system for measuring whole body vibration, by definition motion in the z direction is _____ to _____. Motion in the y direction is _____ to _____. And motion in the x direction is _____ to _____.**

Head to toe.
Side to side (shoulder to shoulder, left to right or right to left).
Front to back (anterior to posterior).

❍   **What anatomic structure is the reference point for segmental (hand-arm) vibration measurements?**

Third metacarpal.

❍   **What occupational standard for whole body vibration is used in the United States?**

ISO 2631, which is identical to ANSI S3.18.

❍   **What occupational standards for segmental (hand-arm) vibration are used in the United States?**

ACGIH-TLV for hand-arm vibration.
ANSI S3.34.
NIOSH no. 89-106 standard for hand-arm vibration.

❍   **What is the goal of the standards for whole body vibration?**

To prevent decreased proficiency and tiring.

OCCUPATIONALLY RELATED CANCER

○ **Increased incidence of what cancer has been associated with women who ingested diethylstilbesterol?**

Breast cancer.

○ **Increased incidence of what cancer has been associated with the daughters of women who ingested diethylstilbesterol?**

Vaginal clear-cell cancer.

○ **What is a thorotrastoma?**

Cancer that has been found at the site of thorotrast extravasation. Thorotrast was a radiologic contrast material used from 1928-1955.

○ **Increased incidence of what cancers have been associated with Thorotrast?**

Thorotrastomas and hepatic angiosarcoma.

○ **Increased incidence of what cancer has been associated with bis (chloromethyl) ether?**

Pulmonary cancer.

○ **Increased incidence of what cancer has been associated with polyaromatic hydrocarbons (PAH)?**

Scrotal cancer.

○ **Increased incidence of what cancer has been associated with beta-napthylamine in dye makers?**

Bladder cancer.

○ **Increased incidence of what cancer has been associated with chromium exposure?**

Pulmonary cancer.

○ **Increased incidence of what cancer has been associated with carbon tetrachloride?** (CCl_4)

Hepatic cancer. *Liver*

(itai-itai "Ouch-Ouch" dz.)

○ **Increased incidence of what cancer has been associated with cadmium?**

Pulmonary cancer. *Lung*

○ **Increased incidence of what cancer has been associated with benzidine?**

Bladder cancer.

○ **Increased incidence of what cancer has been associated with anabolic steroids?**

Hepatic adenoma and, possibly, angiosarcoma and hepatocellular carcinoma. *Liver*

○ **Increased incidence of what cancer has been associated with aflatoxins?**

Hepatic cancer. *Liver*

○ **Increased incidence of what cancer has been associated with vinyl chloride?**

Hepatic angiosarcoma. *of Liver*

○ **Increased incidence of what cancer has been associated with cigarette smoke?**

Pulmonary cancer. *Lung*

○ **Increased incidence of what cancer has been associated with exposure to Agent Orange (TCDD)?**

Soft tissue sarcoma, non-Hodgkin's lymphoma, and Hodgkin's disease.

○ **Increased incidence of what cancer has been associated with exposure to berrylium?** *(Be)*

Pulmonary cancer. *Lung*

○ **Increased incidence of what cancer has been associated with inhalation of nickel?**

Pulmonary cancer. *Lung*

○ **Increased incidence of what cancer has been associated with benzene?**

Acute myelogenous leukemia (AML).

Inorganic

○ **Increased incidence of what gastrointestinal cancer has been associated with arsenic?**

Arsenic → Lung, Liver, Bladder, Skin CA.

Hepatic angiosarcoma. *Liver*

○ **Increased incidence of what genitourinary cancer has been associated with arsenic?**

Bladder cancer.

○ **Increased incidence of what skin cancers have been associated with arsenic?**

Squamous cell, basal cell and Bowen's disease.

○ **Increased incidence of what cancer has been associated with chronic copper exposure (the Bordeaux mixture)?**

Pulmonary cancer and hepatic angiosarcoma. *Lung + Liver*

○ **Increased incidence of what cancer has been associated with formaldehyde?**

Nasopharyngeal carcinoma.

○ **What is an initiator?**

A substance the produces a mutation.

○ **What is a promoter?**

A substance that does not produce a mutation, but completes the neoplastic transformation usually by altering gene expression and inducing neoplastic growth of cells.

○ **Is benzo(a)pyrene a promoter or an initiator?**

Promoter.

○ **Increased incidence of what cancer has been associated with occupational exposure to asbestos?**

Pulmonary mesothelioma.

○ **Increased incidence of what cancer has been associated with chewing Betel nut?** */or chewing tobacco*

Oral cancer.

○ **Increased incidence of what cancer has been associated with radon?** Rn^{222}

Pulmonary cancer. *Lung*

○ **Increased incidence of what cancer has been associated with chewing tobacco?**

*   *IARCC*   1 Carcinogenic to humans
2 a probable
2 b possible
3 Not classified
4 not carcinogenic

Oral cancer.

O   **What is the meaning of an IARCC (<u>International Agency for Research on Cancer Carcinogen Designations</u>) designation of 1?**

There is sufficient evidence that the substance is carcinogenic to humans.

O   **What is the meaning of an IARCC (International Agency for Research on Cancer Carcinogen Designations) designation of 2a?**

Probably carcinogenic to humans. There is either limited human data or sufficient animal data of carcinogenicity.

O   **What is the meaning of an IARCC (International Agency for Research on Cancer Carcinogen Designations) designation of 2b?**

Possibly carcinogenic to humans. There is limited evidence in humans and no sufficient evidence in animals of carcinogenicity.

O   **What is the meaning of an IARCC (International Agency for Research on Cancer Carcinogen Designations) designation of 3?**

Not classifiable as to its carcinogenicity to humans.

O   **What is the meaning of an IARCC (International Agency for Research on Cancer Carcinogen Designations) designation of 4?**

Probably not carcinogenic to humans.

O   **What cancer has been associated with the commercial fishing industry?**

Dermal (from ultraviolet light).

O   **What cancer has been associated with the <u>insulation industry</u>?**

Pulmonary cancer (from asbestos). *Lung*

O   **What cancer has been associated with the <u>petroleum industry</u>?**

Pulmonary cancer (from polycyclic hydrocarbons).

O   **What cancer has been associated with the <u>shipbuilding industry</u>?**

Pulmonary cancer (from asbestos).

○ **What does the Ames test determine?**

Mutagenicity.

○ **CEA (carcinoembryonic antigen) is a bio-marker for what cancers?**

~~Breast~~ and colorectal.

○ **CA 125 is a bio-marker for what cancer?**

~~Breast.~~ *Ovarian*

○ **PSA (prostate specific antigen) is a bio-marker for what cancer?**

Prostate.

○ **Alpha fetoprotein is a bio-marker for what cancers?** *(also β-hCG, CA19-9)*

Testicular, liver and pancreatic.

OCCUPATIONAL EPIDEMIOLOGY

○   **The observation that complicated, confounded disease is more likely to be referred to a specialist or a specialized center and subsequently be described in the literature than is less confounded disease is known as _____.**

Berkson's paradox.

○   **What is the study of how disease is distributed in populations?**

Epidemiology.

○   **What term describes the prevention of disease in people who are well and do not have the disease in question?**

Primary prevention.

○   **List 2 examples of primary prevention.**

Immunization, personal protective equipment (PPE), condom use, health education

○   **What term describes the prevention of morbidity through identification of disease at an early stage, facilitating early intervention?**

Secondary prevention.

○   **Name the components of the epidemiologic triad.**

Agent (toxin, drug, virus, bacteria, etc.).
Environment.
Host (individual, population, etc.).

○   **The routine ("normal") presence of a disease within a particular geographic area is defined as _____.**

Endemic.

○   **If a disease occurs in a given geographic region or population at a higher rate than expected, that disease is said to be ____.**

Epidemic.

○   **Name the term that describes a worldwide epidemic.**

Pandemic.

○   **The number of new cases of a disease divided by the population at risk during a specified period of time is known as _____.**

Incidence.

○   **The number of persons** *(existing cases)* **with disease at a specified time divided by the number of persons in the population at that same time is known as _____.**

Prevalence.

○   **Which measure of morbidity (incidence or prevalence) can be used as a measure of risk?**

Incidence.

○   **Which measure of morbitidity (incidence or prevalence) represents the burden of disease in the population and, therefore, is a tool for planning health services?**

Prevalence.

○   **In a steady-state scenario, what is the relationship between disease incidence, disease prevalence, and duration of disease?**

Prevalence = Incidence x Duration of disease
(Assumptions: stable rates, in-migration = out-migration)

○   **What term describes the total number of deaths from all causes in one year divided by midyear population?**

Annual death rate or annual mortality rate.

○   **A mortality rate is a good estimate of disease incidence when the duration of disease is (long or short).**

Short.

○   **What is the difference between mortality rate and case fatality rate?**

In case fatality rate, the numerator includes only those people dying of the disease of interest and the denominator includes only those people who have the disease of interest. In mortality rate, the denominator includes the entire population, even those free of disease.

○ **Fetal mortality is the number of stillbirths per 1000 births of gestational age greater than __ weeks.**

28.

○ **Which term describes the number of deaths in the first 28 days of life per 1000 live births in one year?**

Neonatal mortality rate.

○ **What term describes the number of deaths under the age of one year per 1000 live births in one year?**

Infant mortality rate.

○ **What term describes the number of deaths between 28 weeks gestation and I week of life per 1000 total births in 1 year?**

Perinatal mortality rate.

○ **Which risk factor is the most important contributor to mortality?**

Older age.

○ **What term describes the observed number of deaths per year divided by the expected number of deaths per year?**

Standardized Mortality Ratio (SMR).

○ **The ability of a screening test to correctly identify those people who have the disease of interest is known as the test's _____.**

Sensitivity.

○ **The ability of a screening test to correctly identify those people who do not have the disease of interest is known as the test's _____.**

Specificity.

○ **This statistic measures the extent that different observers agree beyond what would be expected by chance alone.**

Kappa statistic.

○ **Of accuracy, precision, validity, and reliability, which pairs are analogous.**

Validity is analogous to accuracy.
Reliability is analogous to precision.

○ **Which study design is the best for evaluating the effectiveness and/or risks of a new treatment modality?**

Randomized trial.

○ **What is the purpose of randomization in a randomized trial?**

To control for potential confounders that are known as well as those that are unknown. To make the intervention group and the control group more comparable.

○ **List 2 methods of masking.**

Use of a placebo.
Blinding of the test subjects.
Blinding of the observers (data collectors and data analysts).

○ **Rate of disease in placebo group) – (Rate of disease in vaccine group)) + (Rate of disease in placebo group) = _____ .**

Efficacy.

○ **(Risk in the exposed group) – (Risk in the unexposed group) = _____ .**

Attributable risk.

○ **(Risk in the exposed group) + (Risk in the unexposed group) = _____ .**

Relative risk. *(RR)*

○ **1 / Attributable Risk = _____ .**

Number Needed to Treat (NNT) to prevent one adverse outcome.

○ **Generalizability = (internal or external) validity**

External validity.

○ **When designing a cohort study, subjects are grouped based on their _____ (exposure or disease) status and then the relationship to the occurrence of _____ (exposure or disease) is explored.**

Exposure.
Disease.

O   **When designing a case-control study, subjects are grouped based on their _____ (exposure or disease) status and then the relationship to the occurrence of _____ (exposure or disease) is explored.**

Disease.
Exposure.

O   **What is the measure of association used when analyzing the results of a cohort study?**

Relative risk.

O   **What is the measure of association used when analyzing the results of a case-control study?**

Odds ratio.

O   **If your study finds an association between exposure and outcome, what guidelines should you consider when determining whether the association is causal?**

Temporal Relationship – did the exposure occur before the disease developed.
Strength of Association – larger relative risk or odds ratio.
Dose-Response Relationship – increased risk of disease with greater exposure.
Replication of the Findings – different studies, different populations.
Biologic Plausibility – does the association make sense.
Alternate explanations have been considered and ruled-out.
Cessation of Exposure – similar to dose-response; decreased disease with decline or elimination of exposure.
Specificity of the Association – a specific exposure is associated with only one disease.
Consistency with other knowledge – similar to replication of findings and biologic plausibility.

O   **What term describes the time duration between exposure and onset of disease?**

Latency.

O   **Cohort studies are easier to conduct when the disease latency is (long or short).**

Short.

O   **A _____ study design is more appropriate when the disease latency is prolonged.** or Dz.is rare

Case-control.

O   **T/F:. In a case-control study design, the control population ideally is the population from which the cases come, not just those people free of disease.**

True.

○ **In a case-control study using sex-matched controls, what will be the odds ratio for the effect of gender on the outcome of interest?**

Odds ratio = 1. Do not match on any variable you may wish to explore in your study. Once you match controls to cases based on sex, you cannot study the relationship between sex and the outcome of interest.

○ **Which study design is characterized by the simultaneous collection of both exposure and outcome data?**

Cross-sectional study.   *(Survey or Prevalence Study)*

○ **The odds ratio is a good approximation of the relative risk when studying (rare or common) diseases.**

Rare.

○ **This term describes how much of the risk of disease can be prevented by eliminating the exposure of interest.**

Attributable risk.

○ **The _____ study design is most appropriate when one wishes to study the association of multiple etiologic factors on the outcome of interest.**

Case-control.

○ **The _____ study design is most appropriate when one wishes to study the association of a single etiologic factor on multiple outcomes of interest.**

Cohort.

○ **What term is used to describe the following phenomenon: When the exposure and outcome data for a group are incorrectly or inappropriately attributed to each individual of that group.**

Ecologic fallacy.

○ **List the 4 types of causal relationships.**

Necessary and sufficient
Necessary but not sufficient
Sufficient but not necessary

Neither sufficient nor necessary

○ **List the three phases of an epidemiological study.**

Design
Data collection
Analysis

○ **What term describes systematic error, during any phase of a study, that affects the internal validity of the study?**

Bias.

○ **Name and describe the effect of data misclassification that is not related to exposure or outcome status.**

Nondifferential misclassification usually results in attenuation of the relative risk or odds ratio toward 1.0.

○ **What is the term used to describe a risk factor that is associated with the exposure of interest and is associated with the outcome of interest, but is not caused by the exposure of interest?**

Confounder.

○ **What are 3 methods that can be used to address the problem of confounding during the design phase of a study?**

Randomizaton.
Matching.
Restriction.

○ **What are 2 methods that can be used to address the problem of confounding during the analysis phase of a study?**

Stratified analysis.
Adjustment/Multivariate analysis.

○ **What is the type of bias that is due to the perception of improved survival only because of earlier diagnosis and not because of delayed death?**

Lead time bias.

○ **What term describes the following phenomenon: Communicable disease outbreaks can be avoided and diseases can potentially be eradicated with less than 100% of the population being immune.**

Herd Immunity.

○ **A public health practitioner is performing _____ _____ when he contacts health care providers to determine the number of new cases of a particular disease rather than waiting for providers to report that same information to the health department.**

Active surveillance.

○ **What term describes the number of live births during a specific time period divided by the mid-period population?**

Crude birth rate.

○ **What term describes the number of live births during a specific time period divided by the mid-period population of women age 15-44 years?**

Fertility rate.

○ **List the steps of an outbreak investigation.**

Verify the diagnosis.
Develop a case definition.
Confirm the existence of an epidemic.
Epidemic curve - Determine the distribution of the cases; person, place, time.
Develop a hypothesis.
Test the hypothesis – statistical tests.
Develop and implement control measures based on conclusions from the data.

○ **What is the difference between efficacy and effectiveness?**

Efficacy is a measure of the treatment's effect under "laboratory" conditions, or ideal conditions. Effectiveness describes the treatment's effect under "real world" conditions.

○ **What are federally mandated councils composed of medical personnel, attorneys, and lay representatives at research institutions that oversee the research conducted at that institution?**

Institution Review Board (IRB).

○ **What term describes the incidence calculation using person-time (patient-years, man-days, etc.) in the denominator?**

Incidence density.

○   **What are the terms that are analogous to epidemic and endemic that describe the transmission of infections from other vertebrates to humans under natural conditions?**

Epizootic and endozootic.

○   **This type of bias refers to overdetection of an outcome because one of the groups in the study is more likely to present to the doctor or have a diagnostic test than the other group.**

Surveillance bias.

○   **What is the difference between a ratio and a proportion?**

With a ratio, there is not necessarily a relationship between the numerator and denominator. With a proportion, the numerator is a subset of the denominator (a rate is a specific type of proportion).

○   **What are 3 sources of demographic data?**

Census.
Sample surveys.
Population registers (Social Security, voter registration, immigration records).

○   **Which type of epidemiologic study is most appropriate for reporting an uncommon presentation of a common disease or a common presentation of an uncommon disease?**

Case Report.

○   **What is the measure of association for a cross-sectional study?**

Prevalence ratio.

○   **What term describes the ongoing, systematic collection, analysis, interpretation, and dissemination of data regarding a health-related event for use in public health action to reduce morbidity and mortality and to improve health?**

Surveillance.

○   **What is the difference between biological monitoring and medical monitoring?**

Biological monitoring involves detecting compounds in the body for the purpose of assessing exposure.
Medical monitoring involves detecting compounds in the body for the purpose of assessing disease.

STATISTICS

○ **What is the relationship between standard deviation and variance?**

SD = ⊕variance $\sigma = \sqrt{variance}$

○ **What is the relationship between standard error and standard deviation?**

SE = SD/⊕n $\frac{SD}{\sqrt{n}}$ or $SE = \frac{\sigma}{\sqrt{n}}$

○ **In a normally distributed population, about ____% of the population lies within the mean + 1 standard deviation. About _____% lies within the mean + 2 standard deviations. About _____% lies within the mean + 3 standard deviations.**

68%
95%
99%

○ **A distribution which is skewed to the left has a tail among the (higher/lower) values being characterized.**

Lower.

○ **Which distribution describes the occurrence of rare events in a large population?**

Poisson distribution.

○ **What named distribution is the distribution of possible outcomes from a series of data characterized by two mutually exclusive categories?**

Binomial distribution.

○ **What term describes the sum of all values in a series divided by the actual number of values in the series?**

Mean.

○ **What term describes the value that divides a series into two equal groups so that half of the values are higher and half are lower?**

Median.

○ **What is the most commonly occurring value in a series of values?**

Mode.

O   **What term describes the difference between the highest and lowest values in a series?**

Range.

O   **What term describes the sum of the squared deviations from the mean divided by the number of the values in the series minus 1?**

Variance.

O   **What term describes the type of methods used to analyze probability values that do not follow a known distribution?**

Nonparametric.

O   **If two events (A and B) are mutually exclusive, then P(A and B) = _____.**

Zero.

O   **The probability of two independent events occurring together, P(A and B) = ____.**

$P(A \text{ and } B) = P(A) \times P(B)$

O   **The probability of only one of two independent events occurring, P(A OR B) = _____.**

$P(A \text{ or } B) = P(A) + P(B) - P(A \text{ and } B)$

O   **If the null hypothesis (Ho) is true/accepted, then any difference detected between the samples or populations being compared is due to _____.**

Chance.

O   **What term describes the type of sampling error that occurs when one rejects a null hypothesis that is actually true (a difference between the groups was detected when a difference actually does not exist)?**

Type I error (α).

O   **What term describes the type of sampling error that occurs when one accepts a null hypothesis that is actually false (one fails to detect a difference that actually exists)?**

Type II error (β).

❍   **What is the relationship between sampling error and the power of a study?**

Power = 1 - β

❋   ❍   **Which statistical test should be used to compare means from sample sizes less than 30?**

Student's t-test.

❍   **How does one calculate degrees of freedom when using the Student's t-test?**

n – 1 or
n1 + n2 – 2

❋   ❍   **Standard error of the mean or standard deviation? Which one is a measure of the accuracy of the sample mean as an estimate of the population mean?**

Standard error of the mean.

❋   ❍   **Standard error of the mean or standard deviation? Which one is a measure of the variability of the observations from a sample of the population?**

Standard deviation.

❋   ❍   **A 95% confidence interval indicates that there is a ___ probability that the population mean lies within the upper and lower confidence limits and a ___ probability that it lies outside these limits.**

0.95
0.05

❋   ❍   **For large samples (n > 30), how does one calculate the upper and lower bounds of a 95% confidence interval?**

Upper bound = point estimate + 1.96 (standard error of the mean)
Lower bound = point estimate - 1.96 (standard error of the mean)

❍   **For r x c contingency table analysis, how does one calculate the degrees of freedom?**

df = (r – 1)(c – 1)
Note: if r = 1 then r – 1 = 1; if c = 1 then c – 1 = 1

❋   ❍   **The chi-square test can only be used if the expected value of each cell in a contingency table is greater than or equal to ___.**

5.

O **The _____ test is used to analyze the data in a 2 x 2 table in which any of the expected values is less than 5.**

Fisher's exact.

O **List the characteristics of a good screening test.**

High sensitivity.
High specificity.
Applicable to a large population.
Acceptable.
Simple.
Harmless.
Inexpensive.

O **What term describes the ability of a screening test to identify correctly those individuals who truly have the disease?**

Sensitivity.

O **What term describes the ratio of the number of individuals with a disease whose screening test is positive to the total number of individuals with the disease who were tested?**

Sensitivity.

O **What term describes the measure of a screening test's ability to correctly identify those individuals who do not have the disease?**

Specificity.

O **What term describes the number of disease-free individuals whose screening test was negative divided by the total number of disease-free individuals who were tested?**

Specificity.

O **What term describes the measure of a screening test's ability to correctly identify those individuals who have the disease among those individuals whose screening test was positive?**

Positive Predictive Value.

O **The positive predictive value of a screening test (increases/decreases) as the prevalence of the disease in the population increases.**

Increases.

○ **Which of the following characteristics of a screening test are influenced by the prevalence of the disease in the population being tested – Sensitivity, Specificity, Positive Predictive Value, Negative Predictive Value.**

Sensitivity and Specificity are independent of disease prevalence.
PPV increases with increasing disease prevalence.
NPV decreases with increasing disease prevalence.

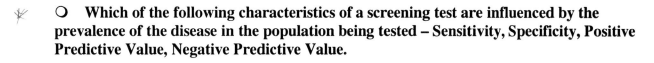

○ **What term describes the ratio of the number of disease-free individuals whose screening test was negative to the total number of individuals who tested negative?**

Negative predictive value.

○ **In a 2 x 3 contingency table, the number of degrees of freedom is ___.**

2.

○ **What is the format of a linear regression equation?**

$y = a + bx$

○ **What term describes the process of testing an individual to find evidence of a disease that is not already being treated?**

Screening.

○ **List the measures of central tendency.**

Mean, median, mode.

○ **List the measures of dispersion.**

Range, variance, standard deviation, coefficient of variation.

○ **What term describes the ratio of the standard deviation of a series to the mean of the series?**

Coefficient of variation [(SD ÷ mean) x 100]

○ **What are 2 statistical tools used to assess the role of chance?**

p-value and confidence interval

O   **The larger the _____, the greater the power to detect a pre-determined difference in risk.**

Sample size.

O   **What term describes the probability of detecting, by chance alone, a difference in risk at least as large at what was observed?**

p-value

O   **What is implied by a 95% confidence interval that includes 1.0?**

A value of 1.0 for the estimate of effect (relative risk or odds ratio) is plausible; therefore, the null hypothesis should be accepted (that is, there appears to be no association between the exposure and outcome of interest).

O   **What term describes a random sample of a population in which individuals are sampled independently, and each individual of the population has the same probability of being selected?**

Simple random sample.

O   **Which sampling technique involves dividing the population into heterogeneous subgroups, then selecting random samples from each subgroup?**

Stratified random sampling.

O   **Which sampling technique involves dividing the population into homogeneous groups based on a given characteristic, then selecting random samples from each group?**

Cluster random sampling.

O   **What is the most common method of analyzing survival data?**

Kaplan-Meier.

O   **Regarding survival analysis, what term describes individuals who did not provide data for the entire observation period (for example, they were lost to follow-up or they entered the study late)?**

Censored observations.

O   **Which statistical test should be used to test the difference between the means of more than 2 independent samples?**

Analysis of Variance (ANOVA).

❍   **How do you standardize a normal distribution for calculations using the standard normal (Z) table?**

You center the distribution at zero by subtracting the mean from every observation. You give the distribution a standard deviation of 1 by dividing all observations by the standard deviation of the original distribution.
$Z = (X - \mu) \div \sigma$

❍   **What is the name of the curve that illustrates graphically how the sensitivity and specificity of a particular test change when different normal/abnormal cutoff points are selected?**

Receiver-Operator Characteristic (ROC) curve.

❍   **Regarding ROC curves, what values are plotted on the x-axis and on the y-axis?**

The y-axis is Sensitivity (0 – 100%).
The x-axis is 1 – Specificity, or False Positive Rate (0 – 100%).

❍   **The ROC curve of a test that is good at discriminating normal from abnormal has what shape?**

The curve crowds the upper left corner of the plot. As the sensitivity is increased, there is little loss of specificity until very high levels of sensitivity are reached.

❍   **If the ROC curve of a test has a favorable profile, how does one use that information to choose the best normal/abnormal cutpoint?**

The best cutpoint is the one closest to the top-left corner of the plot.

❍   **When comparing the ROC curves of 2 different tests, the better test has ____ (more or less) area under the curve than the poorer test.**

More.

❍   **Even if a population has a non-normal distribution, the sample means from repeated samples from this distribution approaches the normal distribution as the sample size increases. This statement describes what mathematical theorem?**

Central Limit Theorem.

❍   **In order for the Central Limit Theorem to apply, the sample size of repeated samples from the parent population must be greater than or equal to ___.**

30.

O The simple linear regression equation is a stochastic (probability) model. The values of the independent variable (X) are under the control of the investigator, but for each value of X, there is a subpopulation of values for the independent variable (Y). These values of Y are generally assumed to have a _____ distribution.

Normal.

O What are the 3 types of data?

Nominal, Ordinal, and Continuous.

O Which type of data can be grouped into categories?

Nominal ~~or categorical~~ data.

O Which type of data can be grouped into categories that can be ranked in a logical order?

Ordinal data.

O Which term describes the type of data that is measured on an arithmetic scale? (The number of potential values for the variable is limited only by the accuracy of the measuring instrument.)

Continuous or interval data.

O The chi square test is most appropriate for analyzing rates and proportions from which type of data?

~~Categorical or~~ *Nominal*

O T/F: A statistically significant result implies that the association or difference is clinically significant.

False.

O What are the 3 quantities that must be set or known in order to calculate the sample size required to perform a study?

The magnitude of the Type I error (α).
The magnitude of the difference the researcher hopes to detect.
The power of the study ($1 - \beta$).

O What is the role of biostatistics in occupational epidemiology?

To determine if the associations between exposures and diseases can be accounted for by chance.

O   **What term describes the natural variation in health outcomes among individuals with similar exposures?**

Chance variation.

O   **Does the p-value alone provide information regarding the magnitude of the effect of exposure?**

No.

O   **What is the non-parametric counterpart of the one-way analysis of variance?** *(oneway ANOVA)*

Kruskal-Wallis test.

O   **What is the non-parametric alternative to the Pearson correlation coefficient?**

Spearman-rho.

O   **What are the nonparametric counterparts to the t-test and paired t-test?**

Wilcoxon and Wilcoxon matched pairs tests.

SILICOSIS

○ **What famous physician reported that miners develop dyspnea on exertion?**

Hippocrates.

○ **Who recognized the relationship between rock dust exposure and dyspnea?**

Ramazzini and Agricola.

○ **Crystaline silica that is unbound to other minerals is referred to as?**

Free.

○ **Bound crystalline silica is referred to as?**

Silicates.

○ **What is the most abundant mineral on earth?**

Silica (silicon dioxide).

○ **What are some examples of silicates?**

Talc, asbestos and kaolin.

○ **Silicosis if a fibrotic lung disease caused by what substance?**

Crystalline silica.

○ **Silica particles of what diameter, are associated with silicosis?**

0.5 to 5 microns.

○ **Silicosis is associated with which specific work settings?**

Mining, quarrying, drilling, tunneling, sandblasting, stonecutting, foundry working.

○ **What is silica chemically?**

Silicon dioxide. (SiO_2)

○ **What is quartz?**

Silicon dioxide.

O   **What are other forms of crystalline silica?**

Cristobalite and tridymite.

O   **What is the range of silica content of various rock formations?**

20-100 percent.

O   **The chronic form of silicosis typically follows what type of exposure?**

Typically decades.

O   **Chronic silicosis often presents with what symptoms and signs?**

Dyspnea on exertion and cough.

O   **Typical radiographic findings of rounded opacities occur in which lung area?**

"eggshell calcifications"

Upper lobes.

O   **The pathologic hallmark of chronic silicosis is?**

Silicotic nodule.

O   **How is the silicotic nodule typically described?**

Cell-free central area surrounded by cellular connective tissue with reticulin fibers.

O   **Chronic silicosis may progress to what process, even after exposure has ceased?**

Progressive massive fibrosis (PMF).

O   **Progressive massive fibrosis is more likely to present with what complaint?**

Exertional dyspnea.

O   **The nodules on chest x-ray of patients with PMF are?**

Greater than 1 centimeter.

O   **The carbon monoxide diffusing capacity capacity is typically what in PMF?**

Reduced.

❍ **Spirometry typically demonstrates what pattern in PMF?**

Restrictive lung disease.

❍ **Recurrent bacterial infections are a possible complication of PMF?**

Yes.

❍ **The differential diagnosis of cavitary lesions and weight loss should also include?**

Tuberculosis.

❍ **Why are pneumothoraces potentially life-threatening in PMF?**

Lung fibrosis makes them difficult to re-expand.

❍ **Cor pulmonale and what are typical terminal events of PMF?**

Hypoxemic respiratory failure.

❍ **Following shorter, yet more intense exposures, what form of silicosis may occur?**

Accelerated silicosis.

❍ **How many years of intense exposure are typically required for the accelerated form?**

5-10 years.

❍ **Clinical features are similar to what form of silicosis?**

Chronic silicosis.

❍ **Lung function deteriorates faster than what form of silicosis?**

Chronic form.

❍ **Patients with the accelerated form typically suffer form what infection?**

Mycobacterial infections.

❍ **Some data suggest that autoimmune disease may be associated with which form of silicosis?**

Accelerated silicosis.

❍ **Acute silicosis may develop within what time period?**

Months to 2 years.

❍ **Symptoms of acute silicosis are often what in comparison to other forms of silicosis?**

More dramatic.

❍ **What is the usual course?**

Rapid progression to respiratory failure.

❍ **Tuberculosis occurs in all three forms of silicosis, but is more common in?**

Accelerated and Acute forms.

❍ **What other associated pulmonary problems may occur?**

Emphysema and bronchitis.

❍ **What type of silica is more injurious?**

Freshly fractured.

❍ **What is the pathogenesis of silicosis?**

Surface properties, including charge, activate macrophages.

❍ **What other uncommon infectious agent may occur in silicosis?**

Nocardia asteroides.

❍ **In endemic areas of tuberculosis, what is the prevalence of TB in silicotics?**

Up to 20 percent.

❍ **What is the first reported symptom?** *of Silicosis*

Shortness of breath.

❍ **What is a common finding in asymptomatic workers?** *of Silicosis*

Abnormal chest radiograph.

❍ **Cough occurs in relation to?**

Chronic bronchitis related to dust inhalation.

○ **How often does hemoptysis occur?**

Rarely.

○ **What should be considered in a silicotic with sudden onset of chest pain?**

Pneumothorax.

○ **How frequently are enlarged hilar lymph nodes encountered?**

5-10 percent of cases of silicotics.

○ **How often does clubbing occur in silicotics?**

Rarely.

○ **According to the ILO Classification, what types of opacifications occur?**

"r" and "q" types.

○ **PMF is characterized by what size of opacities?**

Large opacities. $(>1 cm.)$

○ **Pleural abnormalities occur?**

Rarely.

○ **What spirometric findings are reported?**

Restriction, obstruction, a mixed pattern.

○ **With distortion of the bronchial tree, what spirometric form predominates?**

Obstruction.

○ **In all forms of silicosis, what spirometric form predominates?**

Obstructive.

○ **What is the correlation between radiographic and ventilatory findings?**

There is a poor correlation.

○ **Is lung biopsy required for diagnosis?**

Only in unusual circumstances.

○ **The International Agency for Research on Cancer (IARC) classifies silica exposure as?**

Group I carcinogen.

○ **What is the mainstay of risk elimination in this illness?**

Prevention of exposure with engineering and PPE controls.

○ **What type of cartridge is indicated for silica exposure?**

HEPA.

○ **Workers have died of silicosis from retaining as little as how much quartz dust?**

1 gram of pure quartz dust.

○ **Workers have died of silicosis from retaining as little as how much tridymite ro cristobalite dust?**

0.5 grams of pure dust.

○ **Wet working has been effective in controlling silicosis in what industries?**

Masons and polishers.

○ **What is the ACGIH TLV-TWA for quartz?**

0.05 mg/m^3.

○ **What is the OSHA PEL-TWA for the total quartz measurement?**

30 mg/m^3 ÷ % SiO$_2$ +2

○ **What is the OSHA PEL-TWA for the total respirable quartz?**

10 mg/m^3 ÷ % SiO$_2$ +2

○ **What is the NIOSH REL-TWA?**

0.05 mg/m^3.

○   **The process of removing sand form molds used in the brass industry has been associated with silicosis. This process is known as?**

Fettled (removing with a hammer and chisel).

○   **Stishovite, a rare crystalline variant, is biologically inert because?**

It lacks the tetrahedral configuration shared by the other forms.

○   **Amorphous forms of silica such as kieselguhr and vitreous silica share what fibrogenic potential?**

Low fibrogenic potential.

○   **In addition to the tetrahedral structure, what factors are important in fibrogenicity?**

Silica particle size and concentration.

○   **What renal manifestations have been described in patients with silicosis?**

Glomerulonephritis, nephrotic syndrome and end-stage renal disease.

○   **What is the propose pathogenesis for the renal injury?**

Immune-mediated mechanisms.

○   **What pro-inflammatory mediator has been suggested to play a role in silicosis?**

Tumor necrosis factor (TNF).

○   **What serologic findings have been reported?**

Positive ANA's and Rheumatoid factors.

TRAUMATIC EMERGENCIES

○ **How does the Occupational Safety and Health Administration (OSHA) define the term occupational injury?**

OSHA defines an occupational injury as "any injury such as a cut, fracture, sprain, amputation, etc., which results from a work-related event or from a single instantaneous exposure in the work environment."

○ **How does the Bureau of Labor Statistics (BLS) of the U.S. Department of Labor (DOL) define the term traumatic injury?**

"A traumatic injury is any unintentional or intentional wound or damage to the body resulting from acute exposure to energy—such as heat or electricity or kinetic energy from a crash—or from the absence of such essentials as heat or oxygen caused by a specific event, incident, or series of events within a single workday or shift." (See separate chapters for questions and answers regarding heat-related illness, cold-related medical problems, and altitude-related illness.)

○ **Are "repetitive stress disorders" considered to be traumatic injuries?**

"Repetitive stress disorders" acquired from work activities are better referred to as "work-related musculoskeletal disorders (MSDs)," which according to the Occupational Safety and Health Administration (OSHA) "are disorders of the muscles, nerves, tendons, ligaments, joints, cartilage and spinal discs. MSDs do not include disorders caused by slips, trips, falls, motor vehicle accidents, or other similar accidents." Moreover, the BLS in its discussion of the term occupational disease (illness) states the following: "An occupational disease is defined as a condition produced in the work environment over a period longer than one workday or shift. Usually an illness is due to repetitive factors over a period of time. It may result from systemic infection, repeated stress or strain, [or] exposure to toxins, poisons, fumes, or other continuing conditions of the environment." Thus, "repetitive stress disorders," more properly termed work-related MSDs, are considered to be illnesses rather than traumatic injuries. (See chapter on musculoskeletal disorders.)

○ **In general, what is the difference between occupational health and occupational safety?**

Occupational health attempts to preserve health and minimize disease (illness); occupational safety attempts to preserve worker safety by minimizing injuries, including traumatic injuries.

○ **One of the basic principles of injury analysis is to separate which two components of an injury?**

The cause of the injury is to be separated from the injury or trauma resulting from the cause (that is, the effect of the cause). Often, interventions can be applied to prevent or minimize injuries from a traumatic event even when the event itself is less amenable to prevention.

❍ **Name differences between "accidents" and "injuries."**

The term "accident" implies lack of identifiable risk factors and lack of liability. It also implies randomness or unpredictability and the idea that the accident is unavoidable. The word "injury" is preferred by many over "accident" because injuries often exhibit predictable patterns, are avoidable, and can be prevented.

❍ **What is the leading cause of years of productive life lost (YPLL) for Americans under the age of 65?**

Injury-related deaths. 35% of all YPLL result from injuries. According to 1990 data, injury-related deaths account for 3.7 million YPLL (to age 65) compared with 1.9 million YPLL for cancer, 1.4 million YPLL for heart disease, and .06 million YPLL for AIDS.

❍ **What element of the U.S. Department of Labor keeps track of occupational illnesses and injuries, and where are these data made available?**

The Bureau of Labor Statistics (BLS) of the U.S. Department of Labor uses its Injuries, Illnesses, and Fatalities (IIF) program to provide these data, which are available at http://stats.bls.gov/iif.

❍ **What program of the BLS records and makes available data on fatal occupational injuries in the U.S.?**

The Census of Fatal Occupational Injuries, or CFOI, which is available online at http://stats.bls.gov/iif/oshcfoi1.htm.

❍ **What program is used by the Centers for Disease Control and Prevention (CDC) to monitor fatal occupational injuries in the U.S.?**

The National Traumatic Occupational Fatalities (NTOF) surveillance system. NTOF data typically report approximately 1,000 fewer deaths per year than do CFOI data.

❍ **What organization within the CDC conducts research into, among other things, traumatic occupational injuries?**

The National Institute for Occupational Safety and Health (NIOSH). See http://www.cdc.gov/niosh/injury.

❍ **Research within NIOSH on traumatic occupational injuries is conducted according to a research strategy developed an interdisciplinary team from NORA. What is NORA, and why is it important to traumatic occupational injuries?**

NORA stands for the National Occupational Research Agenda. One of its identified research priorities is traumatic occupational injuries. NORA also schedules NOIRS, or National Occupational Injury Research Symposia.

O   **NIOSH offers an onsite program designed to provide data on investigations of fatal occupational injuries. What is the name of this program?**

The NIOSH Fatality Assessment and Control Evaluation (FACE) Website, which can be found at http://www.cdc.gov/niosh/face/faceweb.html.

O   **The National Center for Injury Prevention and Control (NCIPC) offers two separate interactive data and statistics systems for providing data on fatal and nonfatal injuries. What are these two programs?**

WISQARS™ (Web-based Injury Statistics Query and Reporting System) and Injury Maps. Information about both is available at http://www.cdc.gov/ncipc/osp/data.htm.

O   **For the year 2000, approximately how many fatalities from acute traumatic injuries were there in private industry?**

Nearly 6,000 (5,915). (There are about 150,000 injury-related deaths annually from all causes of injuries in and out of the workplace.) Between

O   **According to CFOI, what were the three most important causes of death from traumatic occupational injuries in the U.S. from 1992 through 2000?**

Highway incidents, homicides, and falls. Highway incidents represented by far the most number of deaths (1,363 in the year 2000). Homicides were the second most numerous type of traumatic occupational fatality from 1992 to 1998, followed by falls; however, in 1999 and 2000, deaths from falls (734 in 2000) outnumbered homicides (677 in 2000).

O   **What types of events or exposures were responsible for the most occupational deaths in 2000?**

Transportation incidents (43% of all occupational fatalities).
Contact with objects and equipment (17%).
Assaults and violent acts (16%).
Falls (12%).
Exposure to harmful substances or environments (8%).
Fires and explosions (3%).

O   **What types of industries in the U.S. provided the most numbers of occupational deaths for the year 2000?**

Construction (1,154).
Transportation (957).

Services (768).
Agriculture (720).
Manufacturing (668).
Retail trade (594).
Government (571).
Wholesale trade (230).
Mining (156).
Finance (79).

O   In what way would it be misleading to characterize construction and transportation as the two most dangerous types of industries for occupational fatalities?

Absolute numbers do not convey risk as much as rates do. In terms of deaths, the most dangerous industries or occupations are those with the highest occupational fatality rates.

O   What types of industries in the U.S. provided the four highest rates of occupational deaths for the year 2000?

Mining: 30.0 deaths per 100,000 workers.
Agriculture: 20.9 deaths/100,000 workers.
Construction: 12.9 deaths/100,000 workers.
Transportation: 11.8 deaths/100,000 workers.

Death rates per 100,000 employees for the other types of industries follow:

- Wholesale trade: 4.3
- Manufacturing: 3.3
- Government: 2.8
- Retail trade: 2.7
- Services: 2.0
- Finance: 0.9

O   What was the average fatality rate for all occupations in the U.S. for the year 2000?

4.3 deaths per 100,000 workers.

O   In terms of occupations, more truck drivers (852) and farm workers (476) died in 2000 than any other single occupation. In 2000, what were the two occupations at highest risk for occupational fatalities?

Timber cutters: 122.1 deaths per 100,000 workers.
Airplane pilots: 100.8 deaths per 100,000 workers.

Rates (deaths per 100,000 workers) for other occupations follow:

- Construction laborers: 28.3

- Truck drivers: 27.6
- Farm workers: 25.1
- Groundskeepers: 14.9
- Laborers (other):   13.2
- Police and detectives: 12.1
- Carpenters: 6.2
- Sales occupations: 2.3

❍   **What three surveillance systems provide data about nonfatal occupational injuries in the U.S.?**

The Survey of Occupational Injuries and Illnesses, or SOII.
The National Electronic Injury Surveillance System (NEISS).
The National Hospital Ambulatory Medical Care Survey (NHAMCS).

(See http://www2.cdc.gov/chartbook/chap4/chartbk4.htm.)

❍   **According to SOII data, about how many nonfatal occupational injuries occurred in the U.S. in 1997?**

About 5.65 million, representing a rate of about 6,600 nonfatal injuries per 100,000 workers. (Injury rates are usually expressed as number of injuries per 100 workers; the use of 100,000 as a denominator in this chapter makes comparisons with fatal injuries easier.)

❍   **NEISS data originate from emergency departments, which presumably do not see all of the occupational injuries recorded by SOII. According to NEISS, what was the average rate for nonfatal occupational injuries treated in U.S. emergency departments in 1998?**

About 2,800 nonfatal injuries per 100,000 full-time workers. These rates can with caution be interpreted as the rates of the more severe occupational injuries in the U.S. for that year.

❍   **Compare the NEISS rates of occupational injuries seen in U.S. emergency departments in 1997 for men with those for women.**

Men have a higher rate of these occupational injuries (3,400 per 100,000 workers) than do women (2,200 per 100,000 workers).

❍   **Compare the NEISS rates of occupational injuries seen in U.S. emergency departments in 1997 for workers aged 20 and over with those for younger workers (16 through 19 years of age).**

Younger workers have higher rates (with a high of 7,800 injuries per 100,000 19-year-old men and 3,900 per 100,000 19-year-old women) compared to older workers (the lowest rates were 1,200 injuries per 100,000 men 75 years old or older and 1,300 injuries per 100,000 women aged

75 or older). (NHAMCS for the highest rates for 1995 through 1997 in male workers 16 and 17 years of age.)

O   **In terms of type of case (cases with restricted activity only, cases without lost workdays, and cases with days away from work), which type of case accounts for both the greatest numbers and also the highest rates of nonfatal occupational injuries?**

Cases without lost workdays represent the most frequent type of case and the highest rate of cases, followed by cases with days away from work and then, with the lowest (but rising) numbers and rates, cases with restricted work only.

O   **Rank the types of private industries in the U.S. by their rates of nonfatal occupational injuries, from the highest to the lowest.**

Transportation and public utilities - about 5,000 nonfatal injuries per 100,000 workers in 1997.
Construction - about 4,500 nonfatal injuries per 100,000 workers in 1997.
Manufacturing - about 4,300 nonfatal injuries per 100,000 workers in 1997.
Agriculture, forestry, and fishing - about 4,000 nonfatal injuries per 100,000 workers in 1997.
Mining -about 3,700 nonfatal injuries per 100,000 workers in 1997.
Wholesale and retail trade - about 3,000 nonfatal injuries per 100,000 workers in 1997.
Services - about 700 nonfatal injuries per 100,000 workers in 1997.

O   **Nonfatal occupational injuries can be classified by type of injury. Name several important types of nonfatal occupational injuries.**

Amputations.
Back, spine, and spinal-cord injuries.
Bruises and contusions.
Cuts (lacerations).
Fractures.
Heat burns and scalds.
Sprains, strains, and tears.

O   **The order of importance of types of nonfatal lost-workday occupational injuries in the U.S. by number of injuries remained remarkably constant during the period 1992 through 1997. By type of injury, rank the preceding list of injury types in descending order of number of cases in the U.S.**

Sprains, strains, and tears - from about 1,000 per year in 1992 to about 800 per year in 1997.
Back, spine, and spinal - cord injuries - from about 650 in 1992 to about 550 in 1997.
Bruises and contusions - about 200 per year.
Cuts/lacerations.
Fractures.
Heat burns and scalds.
Amputations.

○ **What category (medical costs, administrative expenses, wage and productivity losses, or employer costs) represents the greatest proportion of economic losses from occupational illnesses and injuries?**

Wage and productivity losses, which for example in Connecticut in 2001 represented 51% of the economic impact from occupational illnesses and injuries. Medical costs represented 18%, administrative expenses 17%, and employer costs 9% of the total economic impact, with fire losses accounting for 3% and motor-vehicle damage accounting for 2%.

○ **What parts of the body are the most frequently injured in work accidents?**

The trunk (about 30% of cases), followed by the fingers and thumbs (about 15% of cases), legs, arms, and hands.

○ **The International Classification of Diseases (ICD) uses more than one kind of code to classify injuries. Contrast ICD N codes with ICD E codes.**

N codes indicate the nature of the injury, that is, the part of the body involved and the type of damage incurred. E codes are so called because they classify injuries according to the external causes of the injuries. They also group injuries by apparent intent (intentional vs. unintentional) and etiology.

○ **Electrocutions, including lightning strikes, affect about 1,500 people per year in the U.S. and kill 100 to 200 people. What workers have by far the highest rate of electrocution in the U.S.?**

Electric linemen, whose rates are more than four times higher than that of electricians, the second-highest group at risk.

○ **Name other workers at high risk for electrocution.**

Construction workers (for whom electrocution is the second highest cause of death), painters, roofers, plumbers, welders using portable arc-welding equipment, miners, agricultural workers, and machinery operators.

○ **List common activities that put workers at risk for electrocution.**

Using portable power tools.
Using faulty power tools, connectors, and electrical outlets.
Using portable arc-welding equipment.
Allowing ladders to contact power lines.
Contacting moisture, including working with wet tools or on damp ground.
Working in irrigation, concrete work, and animal slaughtering, where water is an important part of the work process.
Wearing inadequate protective clothing.
Working with irrigation pipes, which may contact power lines.

US Households:
AC, 60 Hz, 110 v

◯ **For a given current flow (amperage), which produces more tissue damage, direct current (DC) or alternating current (AC)?**

Alternating current (AC).

◯ **What is Ohm's law?**

Resistance (in ohms) = voltage (in volts) / current flow, or amperage (in amps).

◯ **The voltage of most household alternating current in the U.S. is 110 volts (110 V), compared to 220 V in Europe. How does this voltage compare to that of a) residential and industrial distribution lines and b) high-voltage lines (between generating stations and distribution transformers) in the U.S.?**

The voltage in typical distribution lines in the U.S. is 7,260 volts, whereas the voltage in high-voltage (high-tension) lines is over 100,000 volts.

◯ **What frequencies of alternating current are the most dangerous to humans?**

Frequencies of 20 to 150 cycles per second, or 20 to 150 Hertz (20-150 Hz).

◯ **Household current in the United States has a typical voltage of 110 volts and a typical frequency of 60 cycles per second (60 cps), or 60 Hertz (60 Hz). Calculate the amperage of this current.**

Insufficient information is given to perform this calculation. For current flow in a wire, the resistance of the wire must be known. For current flow in a body in the path of an electrical current, the resistance of the body must be known.

◯ **The resistance of skin to a given current varies widely depending upon many factors, including skin thickness, the numbers of follicles in the skin, whether cuts or abrasions are present, and how much moisture is present. For example, the resistance of a dry hand holding a wire may be 15,000 to 50,000 ohms, whereas the resistance of wet skin to the same applied voltage may be only 3,000 to 6,000 ohms. Skin resistance to alternating current is also less than resistance to direct current. Why?**

Alternating current induces alternating magnetic fields that readily penetrate the body and make skin resistance only a very minor factor in the ability of an AC current to induce current flow in the body.

◯ **Under typical conditions, what voltages of applied current can cause death in humans?**

Voltages of 25 volts or greater are potentially lethal; two fatalities involved applied voltages of 46 and 60 volts.

○   **Compare the threshold of perception (the minimal flow detectable as a tingling sensation) for alternating current at a frequency of 60 cycles per second (60 Hertz, or 60 Hz) to the threshold of perception for direct current.**

The threshold of perception for AC at 60 Hz is one to two milliamperes (1-2 mA), whereas the threshold of perception for DC is 5 mA.

○   **After alternating current has reached a certain value, current-induced tetany prevents hands that have grasped a wire from releasing the wire voluntarily. Compare this "let-go" threshold for AC to the "let-go" threshold for DC.**

The maximal current that can be grasped while still retaining the ability to open the hands and voluntarily release a grip on the conducting wire is about 15 mA for AC and about 75 mA for DC. Current thresholds are usually slightly higher for men than for women.

○   **Since electrical current flowing through a hand and arm would presumably induce tetany in both flexor and extensor muscles, why does flexion predominate?**

Two possible reasons suggest themselves: a) The flexors are stronger than the extensors; b) when hands grasp a wire, the current on its way through the body may flow more directly through the flexors in the forearm than through the extensors.

○   **What is the relationship of skin resistance to electrical burns of the skin?**

Greater skin resistance means that more heat is dissipated as the current passes through the skin. This so-called joule heating means that skin with higher resistance affords more protection to the passage of current into the body, but at the cost of suffering burns. When resistance is lowered and diffused by the presence of moisture or by immersion, current may penetrate the body without leaving any burn marks at all.

○   **In reference to electrical burns, what is the relevance of plasma and arcing?**

Electrical current near or in contact with the skin may raise the local temperature so high (2,500° to 10,000° C, or about 4,500° to 18,000° F) that an arc is formed by conversion of atoms in the body to plasma, which as a separate state of matter refers to an electrically neutral gas-like collection of high-energy ions, electrons, and other particles. With voltages under about 300 volts, direct contact must be made with the current; with higher voltages, the arc may form (from the skin, not in the air) even when a gap exists between the current source and the body. The high temperatures involved superheat the surrounding air and create sound that ranges from the crackle of a welding arc to the thunderclap of a lightning strike. The pressure wave associated with lightning arcs can propel victims against objects, resulting in blunt or penetrating trauma. Plasma can also be generated from electrical power lines in contact with the body and may result in condensation of metal on the skin to form an electroplating-like coating.

○   **What is the usual mechanism of death in electrocution?**

Cardiac dysrhythmias (either asystole or ventricular fibrillation), respiratory arrest (either from muscle tetany or from muscle failure), or both. High voltages passing through the head may also cause permanent brain damage (via hemorrhage, infarction, and cerebral edema) and central apnea (from failure of the respiratory center in the medulla).

○   **With alternating current of 60 Hz and 110 volts (i.e., standard household current in the U.S.), what applied amperage leads to ventricular fibrillation?**

This depends upon the duration of the applied current. For a current duration of ten milliseconds (10 msec), 500mA is required to produce ventricular fibrillation. The relationship between current duration and fibrillation ventricular is neither linear nor logarithmic; thus, increasing the current duration tenfold from 10 msec to 100 msec decreases the fibrillation threshold to 400 mA, but increasing the duration another order of magnitude, to one second, reduces the threshold to 50 mA. When current is applied for greater than three seconds, 40 mA suffices to cause ventricular fibrillation.

○   **List other pathophysiological effects of electrocution.**

There is often thrombosis in blood vessels that serve as carriers of current, and there may be muscle necrosis as well. Destruction of muscle may lead to myoglobinuria and acute tubular necrosis, as in a crush injury. Additional injuries can be sustained from falls or other movements secondary to tetanic muscle contraction.

○   **What is keraunoparalysis (Charcot's paralysis)?**

A usually self-limited electrical injury (from high-voltage lines or from lightning) that causes paresthesias, pain, cold, weakness, and pulselessness in one or more extremities. The signs and symptoms mimic those of compartment syndrome, although most cases resolve spontaneously.

○   **What is a typical Lichtenberg figure and how serious is it?**

The characteristic feather-like pattern of erythema that sometimes develops within hours of a lightning strike and typically resolves within a day. Rather than a true burn, it represents the delayed manifestation of a shower of electrons and does not need treatment.

○   **What is lightning standstill and why is it important?**

Lightning standstill refers to a state of quasi-suspended animation that appears to occur from a lightning strike. With lightning standstill, cellular decay is arrested for a time even though breathing and circulation may cease. For this reason, resuscitation of apparently dead lightning-strike victims even after several minutes of apnea and pulselessness has been successful and should always be attempted.

❍   **Why may the use of traditional formulas (e.g., the Brooke or Parkland formulas) for fluid replacement in burn patients quite possibly underestimate fluid requirements in victims of electrical burns?**

Because of additional damage sustained to deep tissues.

❍   **Head injuries comprise about what percentage of work injuries?**

About 4%.

❍   **Injuries to the scalp tend to bleed profusely. Why?**

Because of the particularly rich blood supply to the network of superficial blood vessels in the dermis of the scalp.

❍   **T/F: Closure of scalp lacerations that have penetrated to the galea aponeurotica should be closed in two layers, with absorbable suture material for the galea and nonabsorbable sutures for the scalp.**

True.

❍   **Apart from the usual ABCs (Airway, Breathing, and Circulation), what is an important assessment to be made in workers with acute head trauma?**

Mental status, particularly level of consciousness. These evaluations should be repeated every 15 to 30 minutes while the patient is under medical observation.

❍   **What is a particularly important symptom to anticipate in workers who have suffered head trauma, and what is its significance?**

From a third to a half of all patients with subarachnoid hemorrhages (SAHs) report an unusual prodromal headache of sudden onset preceding the actual hemorrhage by days to weeks. The headache is severe, often described as the worst headache of the patient's life; and it may be accompanied by nausea and vomiting. Such headaches are often misdiagnosed as migraine headaches, sinusitis, or even malingering; but they probably represent minor leaking of blood into the subarachnoid space and are therefore often called "warning leaks" or "herald bleeds." Workers who have suffered head trauma need to be warned to seek medical attention promptly should this kind of a headache occur.

❍   **Fixed and dilated pupils are a grave prognostic sign following acute head trauma and often indicate brainstem compression. What would fixed and constricted pupils in this situation suggest?**

Hemorrhage into the pons.

❍ **What changes in vital signs are classically associated with an acute rise in intracranial pressure following head trauma?**

A rise in systolic blood pressure while the diastolic blood pressure drops or remains the same.
Bradycardia.
Irregular breathing.
Fever.

❍ **What clinical findings in a head-trauma victim suggest a basilar skull fracture?**

Periorbital ecchymoses ("raccoon eyes"), ecchymoses behind the ear (Battle's sign) (after 8 to 12 hours), leakage of cerebrospinal fluid from the nose or ear (CSF rhinorrhea or otorrhea), and blood behind the tympanic membrane (hemotympanum),

❍ **In addition to cervical-spine radiographs and plain films of the skull, which of the following two studies should be done in a head-trauma patient, computerized tomography (CT) or magnetic resonance imaging (MRI)?**

Computerized tomography (CT) of the head. MRI is not suited to detecting acute hemorrhage in head-trauma victims.

❍ **What are the two most common fractures of the face?**

Nasal fractures, following by mandibular fractures.

❍ **Fractures of the maxilla usually involve the transfer of large amounts of energy. What is the Le Fort classification of maxillary fractures?**

A Le Fort I fracture is a transverse fracture of the maxilla superior to the teeth.
A Le Fort II fracture is a fracture that extends superomedially from the lateral aspects of the maxilla through the infraorbital plates to the bridge of the nose.
A Le Fort III fracture is a complex craniofacial disruption involving fractures of the maxilla, infraorbital rims, and zygoma.

❍ **What radiological view is usually used to demonstrate a "blowout" fracture of the orbital floor?**

A Waters view.

❍ **According to the Occupational Medicine Practice Guidelines of the American College of Occupational and Environmental Medicine (ACOEM), what are the warning signs ("red flags") for possible cervical fracture following head or neck trauma?**

From the medical history:
- Direct blow to the head.
- Excessive force to the neck, with pain after the injury.

- Loss of consciousness.
- Ejection from a vehicle.

From the physical examination:
- Pain sufficient to prevent the patient from moving his or her neck.
- Severe tenderness over the midline of the cervical vertebrae.
- Observation that the patient is holding his or her head for stability.
- Neurological deficits.

○ **According to the Occupational Medicine Practice Guidelines of the American College of Occupational and Environmental Medicine (ACOEM), what are the warning signs ("red flags") for possible cervical-spinal-cord compromise following acute head or neck trauma?**

From the medical history:

- Significant trauma to the neck.
- Paresthesias involving the upper (with or without the lower) extremities.
- Weakness of the upper or lower extremities.
- Global weakness of the upper extremities.
- Difficulty walking.

From the physical examination:
- Severe spasm of neck muscles.
- Weakness of major muscle groups in the upper or lower extremities.
- Bilaterally decreased sensation in the upper or lower extremities.
- Disturbance of bowel or bladder control.
- Positive Babinski signs.
- Hyperactive reflexes.

○ **According to the Occupational Medicine Practice Guidelines of the American College of Occupational and Environmental Medicine (ACOEM), what are the physical-examination warning signs ("red flags") for rapidly progressive neurological compromise following acute traumatic injury to the shoulder?**

Decreased sensation, reflexes, or strength in the upper extremities.

○ **According to the Occupational Medicine Practice Guidelines of the American College of Occupational and Environmental Medicine (ACOEM), what are the physical-examination warning signs ("red flags") for rapidly progressive vascular compromise in a patient with acute shoulder pain?**

Decreased pulses in the upper extremity.
Cold and absent pulses in the upper extremity.
Pain-free full range of motion.
Differences in blood-pressure measurements between the upper extremities.

Bruit (with a thoracic aortic aneurysm).

○   **According to the Occupational Medicine Practice Guidelines of the American College of Occupational and Environmental Medicine (ACOEM), what are the warning signs ("red flags") for acute rotator-cuff tear in a young worker?**

From the medical history:
- Heavy lifting.
- Sudden pulling.
- Pain in the shoulder with overhead work.
- Weakness on elevation and external rotation.

From the physical examination:
- Weakness of abduction with thumbs down.
- Weakness of external rotation.
- Bilaterally decreased sensation in the upper or lower extremities.
- Weakness on tests of the supraspinatus and infraspinatus muscles.

○   **According to the Occupational Medicine Practice Guidelines of the American College of Occupational and Environmental Medicine (ACOEM), what are the warning signs ("red flags") for elbow fracture?**

From the medical history:
- History of significant trauma.
- A fall onto an outstretched hand.

From the physical examination:
- Disturbance in the triangular relationship involving the olecranon and the epicondyles.
- Significant bruising, if subacute.

○   **According to the Occupational Medicine Practice Guidelines of the American College of Occupational and Environmental Medicine (ACOEM), what are the warning signs ("red flags") for rapidly progressive neurological compromise following acute traumatic injury to the forearm, wrist, or hand?**

From the medical history:
- Rapidly progressive numbness, paresthesias, or weakness in the distribution of the radial, median, or ulnar nerves.

From the physical examination:
- Sensory deficits in the distribution of the radial, median, or ulnar nerves.
- Loss of grip strength while attempting to pick up objects.
- Progressive atrophy.

○   **According to the Occupational Medicine Practice Guidelines of the American College of Occupational and Environmental Medicine (ACOEM), what are the warning signs ("red** flags") for rapidly progressive vascular compromise following acute traumatic injury to the forearm, wrist, or hand?

From the medical history:
- A history of vascular disease.
- A history of diabetes.
- A hand that feels cold to the patient.

From the physical examination:
- Decreased pulses.
- Decreased capillary filling.
- A hand that is cool to the touch or pale.

○ **According to the Occupational Medicine Practice Guidelines of the American College of Occupational and Environmental Medicine (ACOEM), what are the warning signs ("red flags") for fracture of the lower spine?**

From the medical history:
- Major trauma, such as a motor-vehicle accident or a fall from a height.
- Minor trauma or strenuous lifting in older or osteoporotic patients.

From the physical examination:
- Severe localized pain over specific spinal processes.
- Percussion tenderness over spinous processes.

○ **What is cauda-equina syndrome (CES)?**

Compression of the nerve roots caudal (distal) to the caudal tip (the conus medullaris) of the spinal cord.

○ **According to the Occupational Medicine Practice Guidelines of the American College of Occupational and Environmental Medicine (ACOEM), what are the warning signs ("red flags") for the cauda-equina syndrome (CES)?**

From the medical history:
- A direct fall or blow involving axial loading.
- Saddle anesthesia.
- Recent onset of bladder dysfunction (e.g., urinary retention, increased frequency, or overflow incontinence).

From the physical examination:
- Unexpected laxity of the bladder or anal sphincter.
- Perianal or perineal sensory loss.
- Major motor weakness in any of the following muscle groups:
  - Quadriceps (knee-extension weakness).
  - Ankle plantar flexors.

- o   Ankle evertors.
- o   Ankle dorsiflexors (foot drop).
- o   Spastic (thoracic) or flaccid (lumbar) paraparesis.
- o   Increased (thoracic) or decreased (lumbar) reflexes.

❍   **What is compartment syndrome?**

Compression of nerves and blood vessels in an anatomic compartment, potentially leading to neurological compromise, vascular compromise, or both.

❍   **According to the Occupational Medicine Practice Guidelines of the American College of Occupational and Environmental Medicine (ACOEM), what are the warning signs ("red flags") for compartment syndrome above or below the knee?**

From the medical history:
- ▪   A history of fracture or other major trauma.
- ▪   A very painful muscular compartment.

From the physical examination:
- ▪   A tense and very tender compartment.
- ▪   Distal signs of neurovascular compromise (signs may be present or absent).

❍   **According to the Occupational Medicine Practice Guidelines of the American College of Occupational and Environmental Medicine (ACOEM), what are the warning signs ("red flags") for neurovascular compromise from acute trauma involving the knee?**

From the medical history:
- ▪   A history consistent with a fracture or a dislocation.
- ▪   A history of peripheral vascular disease.
- ▪   A history of diabetes.
- ▪   Pain or pallor at or below the knee.

From the physical examination:
- ▪   Decreased or absent popliteal or pedal pulses.
- ▪   Pale and cold skin distal to the knee.
- ▪   Paralysis of the distal lower extremity.
- ▪   Painless swelling of the knee (Charcot's joint).

❍   **What industry divisions in the U.S. have the highest rates of work-related homicides?**

Service industries, transportation, and handlers and laborers.

❍   **What occupations and workplaces in the U.S. have the highest rates of work-related homicides?**

Taxicab drivers and chauffeurs, sheriffs and related officials, and police and detectives.

○ **In general, are women or men in the U.S. at higher risk of dying as the result of intentional injuries incurred at work?**

Women.

○ **What age group is the most vulnerable to work-related homicides?**

Older workers (those 65 years of age and older), especially part-time cooks, bartenders, security guards, and managers or supervisors of hotels and motels.

○ **Although many studies of homicide in the workplace do not include data on the time of day of the attacks, what part of the day seems to be the dangerous in terms of the risk of work-related homicide?**

Late afternoon, evening, and late at night, particularly from 10 p.m. to 2 a.m.

○ **T/F: Robberies represent a greater risk for workplace homicide than do acts by disgruntled workers.**

True. Robbery accounts for about 75% of work-related homicides compared to about 10% perpetrated by work associates and about 5% each from police killed in the line of duty, security guards killed while working, and employees killed by personal acquaintances (including relatives).

○ **List risk factors for work-related homicide involving retail workers.**

Exchanging money with the public.
Working alone or in small numbers.
Working late at night or early in the morning.
Working in high-crime areas.

○ **What kinds of weapons are most frequently employed in workplace homicides?**

Firearms show an overwhelming preponderance over all other methods.

○ **The Occupational Safety and Health Administration (OSHA) has categorized workplace violence into three types. What are they, and what percentages of homicides does each type represent?**

Type I (60%) is external (e.g., attacks by people, usually criminals, from outside the organization).
Type II (30%) is service-related.
Type III (10%) is internal (e.g. by disgruntled or troubled employees).

○ **Several models have been used to analyze traumatic injuries in the workplace. The Suchman model considers four aspects of a workplace injury. What are these four characteristics?**

a) Predisposing characteristics:
- Susceptibility.
- Hazardous environment.
- Agent.

b) Situational Characteristics:
- Risk taking.
- Appraisal of the hazard.
- Margin of error.

c) Conditions.
- Unexpected.
- Unavoidable.
- Unintentional.

d) Effect.
- Injury.
- Damage.

○ **The Gordon epidemiological model of traumatic injuries in the workplace focuses on the three aspects of the preventive-medicine/public-health triad. What are threes three elements?**

Agent, environment, and host.

○ **The Haddon matrix, perhaps the best-known method of analyzing acute injuries, is based upon an approach to motor-vehicle injuries. It involves construction of a matrix using three groups of three aspects each. Name the groups and the subdivisions of each group.**

a) Time sequence (phases):
- Precrash.
- Crash.
- Postcrash.

b) Crash factors:
- Human.
- Vehicle.
- Environment.

c) Crash losses:
- People.

- Vehicles.
- Environment.

(Because of the rough equivalence of the subcategories of b) and c), the matrix is usually constructed by listing the subcategories of a) along one side of the matrix and using b) and c) to label the top and bottom, respectively, of the matrix.)

○ **What are Haddon's ten countermeasures, which use an energy-transfer model of injury, as applied to acute traumatic emergencies in the workplace?**

1) Prevent the initial marshaling of the form of energy (e.g., dismantle dangerous machinery).
2) Reduce the amount of energy marshaled (e.g., reduce the amount of explosive in construction).
3) Prevent the release of energy (e.g., use a retaining wall to prevent mudslides).
4) Modify the rate of spatial distribution of release of energy from its source (e.g., eliminate utility poles from the sides of roadsides in work areas).
5) Separate in time or space the energy being released from the susceptible structure (e.g., use fire escapes).
6) Separate the energy being released from the susceptible structure by interposition of a material barrier (e.g., use hardened glass fume-hood windows).
7) Modify the contact surface, subsurface, or basic structure that can be impacted (e.g., add energy-absorbing seats to the interior of a vehicle).
8) Strengthen the living or nonliving structure that might be damaged by the energy transfer (e.g., institute worker conditioning).
9) Move rapidly to detect and evaluate damage to counter its continuation and extension (e.g., activate first responders; use basic-life-support techniques).
10) Use all those measures (including intermediate and long-term reparative and rehabilitative measures) that fall between the emergency period following the damaging energy exchange and the final stabilization of the process (e.g., use skin grafts for burn victims).

○ **Group Haddon's ten countermeasures into pre-incident, incident, and post-incident phases.**

Interventions 1 through 3 apply to the pre-incident phase, interventions 4 though 8 apply to the incident phase, and interventions 9 and 10 apply to the post-incident phase.

○ **What is the hazard against which lock-out, tag-out was designed?**

Officially, "hazardous energy" from the inadvertent activation of a device.

○ **What is the difference between lockout (and a lockout device) and tagout (and a tagout device)?**

The official OSHA definitions are as follows:

"Lockout." The placement of a lockout device on an energy isolating device, in accordance with an established procedure, ensuring that the energy isolating device and the equipment being controlled cannot be operated until the lockout device is removed.

"Lockout device." A device that utilizes a positive means such as a lock, either key or combination type, to hold an energy isolating device in the safe position and prevent the energizing of a machine or equipment. Included are blank flanges and bolted slip blinds.

"Tagout." The placement of a tagout device on an energy isolating device, in accordance with an established procedure, to indicate that the energy isolating device and the equipment being controlled may not be operated until the tagout device is removed.

"Tagout device." A prominent warning device, such as a tag and a means of attachment, which can be securely fastened to an energy isolating device in accordance with an established procedure, to indicate that the energy isolating device and the equipment being controlled may not be operated until the tagout device is removed.

○   **Psychological sequelae of traumatic emergencies are important causes of lost work time and losses in productivity. Symptoms of posttraumatic stress disorder (PTSD) may occur immediately after a traumatic emergency. Can the diagnosis of PTDS be made at that time?**

No; to meet the criteria of the Diagnostic and Statistical Manual IV (DSM-IV), symptoms must be present for at least a month before the diagnosis of PTSD can be made.

○   **PTSD may be the result of a single acute traumatic emergency. However, it may also follow a series of lesser incidents. Although there is no official DSM-IV name for the cumulative kind of PTSD, what is the suggested term for this condition?**

Complex PTSD.

○   **Following a physical assault, who is at greater risk for developing PTSD, men or women?**

Women.

○   **Following acute traumatic emergencies associated with natural disasters, accidents, or death of a loved one, who is at greater risk of developing PTSD, men or women?**

Under these circumstances there appears to be no difference in PTSD rates between men and women.

○   **What early psychological symptoms following an acute traumatic emergency predispose to the eventual development of PTSD?**

Symptoms of dissociation, avoidance, or numbing (as contrasted with hyperarousal).

MUSCULOSKELETAL

○ **Raynaud's phenomenon occurs as part of a syndrome called _____, which is seen in workers exposed to vinyl chloride.**

Acroosteolysis.

○ **The hallmark of this disease is the triad of Raynaud's phenomenon, scleroderma-like skin lesions on the hands and arms, and lytic bone lesions of the terminal phalanges.**

Acroosteolysis.

○ **Which syndrome is characterized by paresthesias, pain, and weakness in the distribution of the median nerve distal to the wrist?**

Carpal Tunnel Syndrome.

○ **Entrapment of the median nerve in the forearm causes _____ _____, which resembles carpal tunnel syndrome but the numbness extends to the forearm.**

Pronator Syndrome.

○ **Which syndrome is characterized by numbness on the ulnar side of the palm and weakness of the hand muscles innervated by the ulnar nerve?**

Cubital Tunnel Syndrome.

○ **Wrist drop can occur as a result of direct pressure to the _____ ____ as it courses the posterior humerus.**

Radial Nerve

○ **Heavy use of the shoulder muscles and hypertrophy of the _____ muscle may cause Thoracic Outlet Syndrome.** (TOS)

Subclavius.

○ **Thoracic Outlet Syndrome may be manifest as intermittent neurovascular insufficiency in the arm resulting from compression of what anatomic structures?**

Brachial Plexus and subclavian artery and/or vein.

O   **Compression of this sensory nerve can cause burning pain and numbness of the lateral thigh.**

Lateral Femoral Cutaneous Nerve.

O   **This nerve may be compressed or injured, leading to foot drop.**

Peroneal Nerve.

O   **Name the clinical syndrome associated with weakness of dorsiflexion, sensory loss on the dorsum of the foot, and sensory loss of the lateral lower leg.**

Foot Drop.

O   **This disorder is characterized by nodular proliferation of fibrous tissue in the palmar fascia accompanied by progressive fixed digital flexion.**

Dupuytren's Contracture.

O   **What is the most common category of work-related illnesses in the United States?**

Work-related musculoskeletal disorders (WMSDs).

O   **List 2 synonyms for work-related musculoskeletal disorder (WMSD).**

Cumulative Trauma Disorder (CTD).
Repetitive Strain Injury (RSI).

O   **List 5 non-occupational risk factors for Carpal Tunnel Syndrome.**

Hypothyroidism, diabetes mellitus, collagen vascular disease, uremia, pregnancy.

O   **Cervical radiculopathy at which level(s) may cause symptoms similar to those of Carpal Tunnel Syndrome.**

C6-C7.

O   **Name the clinical sign in which an electric shock-like feeling occurs in the fingers after tapping the palmar surface of the wrist.**

Tinel's sign.

O   **What is the clinical test that attempts to reproduce paresthesias after 1 minute of wrist flexion?**

Phalen's test.

○   **Atrophy of which group of muscles in the hand is highly suggestive of advanced or severe Carpal Tunnel Syndrome.**

Thenar atrophy.

○   **What term describes a soft, round structure, usually over the dorsum of the wrist and usually connected to underlying joints or tendons?**

Ganglion.

○   **This term describes an injury of a muscle, ligament, or tendon in which the normal range of motion of the tissue has been exceeded due to lifting a heavy weight or bearing an external force. None of the tissue fibers have been torn.**

Strain.

○   **This term describes an injury of a ligament resulting in torn fibers, inflammation, and edema.**

Sprain.

○   **Define the term: Third-degree sprain.**

Complete tear of a ligament.

○   **This term describes inflammation of a tendon.**

Tendinitis.

○   **This term describes inflammation of a tendon sheath.**

Tenosynovitis.

○   **What is the most common musculoskeletal complaint in the workplace?**

Occupational back pain.

○   **List 3 risk factors for occupational low back pain.**

Heavy repetitive lifting, pushing, or pulling.
Exposure to industrial or vehicular vibration.
History of previous back injury and/or non-back injury claims.
Job dissatisfaction.
Cigarette smoking.
Poor ratings from supervisors.

Repetitive boring tasks.
Younger age.
Shorter duration of employment.

❍ **Chronic back pain refers to back pain refractory to conservative measures and present for over ___ weeks.**

6.

❍ **List at least 3 causes of low back pain.**

Muscle or ligament injury.
Vertebral fracture.
Degenerative disk disease or degenerative arthritis.
Spinal stenosis.
Anomolies of vertebral anatomy (example: spondylolisthesis).
Herniated nucleus pulposis (HNP) of intervertebral disks.
Systemic diseases (examples: cancer, infection, ankylosing spondylitis).
Abdominal disorders not related to the spine.

❍ **What are the NIOSH criteria for diagnosis of Carpal Tunnel Syndrome?**

Symptoms suggestive of carpal tunnel syndrome.
Objective findings consistent with carpal tunnel syndrome (Tinel's sign, Phalen's sign, decreased sensation in median nerve distribution, abnormal nerve conduction/EMG across the carpal tunnel).
Evidence of work-relatedness.

❍ **What is the term describing osteophytes of the distal interphalangeal (DIP) joints due to osteoarthritis of the hands?**

Heberden's nodes.

❍ **What is the term describing osteophytes of the proximal interphalangeal (PIP) joints due to osteoarthritis of the hands?**

Bouchard's nodes.

❍ **Regional musculoskeletal disorders caused by nerve entrapment have characteristic clinical features. List 3 of these clinical features.**

Dysesthesias are localized to the sensory distribution of the nerve.
Paresthesias and pain are more pronounced at rest than with use.
Motor deficit is a late finding. Sensory fibers are more sensitive to insult.
Tinel's sign is common clinical finding.
EMG and nerve conduction studies are the gold standard for diagnosis.

○ **Which gender is at higher risk of developing carpal tunnel syndrome?**

Female.

○ **What is the main cause of back injury in health care workers?**

Patient handling.

○ **List 3 occupations at high risk for developing carpal tunnel syndrome.**

Meat, fish, and poultry processing.
Sewing machine operation (garment workers).
Leather tanning.
Manufacturing (both heavy and light).
Forestry workers.
Grocery checkers.
Dental hygienists.
Musicians.

○ **List 3 workplace stressors that have been associated with the development of carpal tunnel syndrome.**

Highly repetitive work.
Forceful hand work.
Hand/wrist vibration.

○ **What are the classic symptoms of carpal tunnel syndrome?**

Numbness, tingling, burning, or pain in at least two of digits 1, 2, or 3 with or without pain in the palm.

○ **What electrodiagnostic findings typically suggest carpal tunnel syndrome?**

Prolonged distal median nerve motor and/or sensory latency.
Slowed conduction velocity in the median nerve across the wrist.
Denervation of the abductor pollicis brevis muscles.

○ **What screening tests should be performed on patients with newly diagnosed carpal tunnel syndrome to look for systemic illnesses associated with CTS?**

Complete blood count.
Blood chemistries (fasting blood sugar, renal function tests).
Erythrocyte sedimentation rate (ESR).
Thyroid stimulating hormone (TSH).
When indicated, serologies for Rheumatoid arthritis and other collagen vascular diseases.

O   **List 3 nonsurgical management options for mild-to-moderate carpal tunnel syndrome.**

Neutral wrist splints at night. *30% effective*
Avoidance of exacerbating ergonomic exposures (occupational and recreational).
Physical therapy and/or occupational therapy for the hand.
Non-steroidal anti-inflammatory agents (NSAIDs).
Corticosteroid injection into the carpal tunnel. *75% effective*

O   **Which nerve can be traumatized by carrying a heavy shoulder pack, causing shoulder pain and winging of the scapula?**

Long thoracic nerve.

O   **What are some of the clinical signs and symptoms of ulnar nerve entrapment at the elbow?**

Forearm pain.
Paresthesias of the fifth finger.
Weakness and atrophy of the hand and forearm muscles.

O   **How do the clinical signs and symptoms differ between ulnar nerve entrapment at the elbow and at the wrist?**

Forearm symptoms (pain and weakness) and signs (weakness and atrophy) are absent when the entrapment is at the wrist.

O   **Entrapment of the peroneal nerve at the fibula can be caused by prolonged squatting. What are the clinical signs and symptoms of this condition?**

Foot drop.
Numbness of the foot.
Paresthesias of the foot.

O   **What term describes low back pain with lower limb symptoms suggesting lumbosacral nerve root compromise?**

Sciatica.

O   **What term describes low back pain without symptoms or signs of lumbosacral nerve root compromise or other serious underlying condition?**

Mechanical low back pain.
Nonspecific low back pain.

○ **What lumbar nerve roots innervate the knee?**

L3 and L4.

○ **In what directions should the knee be stressed in order to evaluate ligamentous stability?**

Varus, valgus, and anterior-posterior.

○ **What are the clinical signs and symptoms of chondromalacia patellae?**

Anterior knee pain with ambulation or while standing from a sitting position.
Pain is worse with walking down stairs rather than upstairs.
Crepitus with passive patellar motion.
Symptoms are reproduced with passive depression of the patella and active flexion of the quadriceps muscle.
Rarely, a joint effusion may be present.

○ **The term internal derangement of the knee describes a tear of which structures?**

Medial meniscus, lateral meniscus.
Anterior cruciate ligament, posterior cruciate ligament.

○ **This condition occurs when snovial fluid from the knee is trapped behind the semimembranous bursae.**

Baker's cyst (synovial cyst).

○ **What term describes entrapment of the ulnar nerve at the elbow?**

Cubital tunnel syndrome.

○ **What is the most common site of ulnar nerve entrapment?**

Elbow (cubital tunnel).

○ **This anatomic space is next to the carpal tunnel; it is bordered by the transverse carpal ligament, the pisiform bone, and the hook of the hammate bone; and it is a site of ulnar nerve entrapment at the wrist.**

Guyon's canal.

○ **What are some conservative measures for managing ulnar nerve entrapment at the elbow?**

Patient education - avoid leaning on the elbows.

Elbow pads.
Ice.
Non-steroidal anti-inflammatory drugs (NSAIDs).

O   **What are the surgical treatment options for ulnar nerve entrapment at the elbow?**

Cubital tunnel release.
Ulnar nerve transposition (from condylar groove to medial forearm).
Medial epicondylectomy.

O   **Radial tunnel syndrome causes pain in what location?**   *(pain with middle finger resistance)*

It causes pain in the extensor muscle mass distal to the lateral epicondyle.

O   **Lateral epicondylitis is characterized by tenderness over the lateral epicondyle and pain with passive flexion of the _____.**

Wrist.

O   **Patients with radial (nerve) *tunnel* syndrome may have had previously unsuccessful treatments for what disorder?**

Lateral epicondylitis.

O   **Pronator syndrome refers to entrapment of the _____ nerve in the forearm?**

Median nerve.

O   **Are wrist splints recommended for relief of the symptoms of pronator syndrome?**

Although both carpal tunnel syndrome and pronator syndrome involve the median nerve, pronator syndrome does not involve nocturnal exacerbation like CTS does.

O   **Which diagnostic study is useful in differentiating between carpal tunnel syndrome and pronator syndrome?**

Nerve conduction. */EMG*

O   **In thoracic outlet syndrome, which type of symptom (neurogenic or vascular) is more common?**

Vascular, due to compromise of the subclavian artery or vein.

O   **What are the known anatomic abnormalities that may cause thoracic outlet syndrome?**

Cervical rib.
Fibrous bands from the transverse process of C7.
Anomolies of the clavicle.
Anomolies of the scalene muscles.

○   **What are the neurogenic symptoms of thoracic outlet syndrome?**

Pain and paresthesias in the medial arm, forearm, and hand.
Diffuse arm pain.
Weakness of the small muscles of the lateral thenar eminence.
Arm fatigue with use.

○   **What are the vascular symptoms of thoracic outlet syndrome?**

Diffuse arm pain.
Fatigue and aching with use.
Coldness.
Weakness.

○   **What term describes inflammation of muscle?**

Myositis.

○   **The most common site of cervical degenerative disk disease is _____.**

C5-6.

○   **Regarding shoulder dislocation, the humeral head most commonly is displaced in which direction?**

Anteriorly.

○   **Describe a positive Finkelstein's test.**

With the thumb grasped in the palm, pain at the first dorsal wrist extensor compartment is elicited with ulnar deviation of the wrist.

○   **What is the likely diagnosis in a patient with pain over the radial side of the thumb, a positive Finkelstein's test, and crepitus over the involved tendon sheath?**

De Quervain's tenosynovitis.

○   **De Quervain's tenosynovitis is classically associated with which overuse injury?**

Overuse of the thumb, repetitive grasping, gripping, cutting.

○ **What is the initial treatment of trigger finger?**

Corticosteroid injection into the synovial sheath at the point of greatest tenderness.

○ **A worker who falls on an outstretched hand and has tenderness in the anatomic snuffbox has _____ until proven otherwise.**

Scaphoid fracture.

IONIZING RADIATION

○ **What is radiation?**

The propagation of energy through space via either electromagnetic waves (electromagnetic radiation) or streams of particles (corpuscular radiation).

○ **What is the difference between ionizing radiation and nonionizing radiation?**

Ionizing radiation is radiation that has sufficient energy to dislodge electrons from atoms, thus creating ions. Nonionizing radiation, also called long-wavelength electromagnetic radiation, does not have sufficient energy to create ions.

○ **In terms of energy, frequency, and wavelength, describe the boundary between nonionizing radiation (long-wavelength electromagnetic radiation) and the short-wavelength component of ionizing radiation.**

A photon energy of 12.4 electron volts (12.4 eV), which is equivalent to 3×10^{12} megahertz (3×10^{12} MHz) and to 100 nanometers (100 nm, or 1×10^{-7} meter). Energies and frequencies above this boundary, and wavelengths below this boundary, constitute ionizing radiation.

○ **Is ultraviolet (UV) radiation ionizing radiation?**

Part of it is. The three bands designated UV-A, UV-B, and UV-C span from 400 nm down to 100 nm (UV-A: 400-315 nm; UV-B: 315-280 nm; UV-C: 280-100 nm). However, ultraviolet radiation technically exists from 400 nm down to 10 nm. The UV radiation between 100 nm and 10 nm has enough energy to ionize atoms. However, the Occupational Safety and Health Administration (OSHA) does not classify ultraviolet radiation as a type of ionizing radiation.

○ **What are the two types of ionizing radiation?**

Particulate radiation (possessing mass and sometimes charge) and short-wavelength (high-energy) electromagnetic radiation, which has neither mass nor charge but exists as waves of associated electric and magnetic forces.

○ **What are the types of particulate ionizing radiation?**

Alpha, beta, neutron, and proton radiation.

○ **What is alpha radiation?**

Ionizing radiation composed of alpha particles, or helium nuclei, each of which has two protons and two neutrons. Streams of alpha particles are also called alpha rays.

❍ What is beta radiation?

Ionizing radiation composed of high-energy beta particles, which may be either negatively charged (alpha particles, or electrons) or positively charged (beta particles, or positrons). Streams of beta particles are also called beta rays.

❍ Do neutrons cause ionization directly?

No; but by colliding with hydrogen nuclei in, for example, water molecules, they can create proton radiation that can ionize other atoms and molecules.

❍ What are the types of nonparticulate (electromagnetic) ionizing radiation?

Gamma radiation, X radiation (X-rays), and ultraviolet radiation between 100 and 10 nm in wavelength.

❍ Describe X-rays.

They are electromagnetic rays that arise from electrons. They include Brehmsstrahlung radiation ("braking radiation"), caused when electrons are suddenly decelerated; and characteristic X-rays, which result when electrons release energy while making transitions to lower energy levels in atoms of heavy metals. Their wavelengths are less than 10 nm, and their frequencies are greater than 3×10^{13} MHz.

❍ Describe gamma rays.

Unlike X-rays, gamma rays are electromagnetic rays that originate from atomic nuclei by interactions between the strong and electromagnetic forces. Their energies overlap with the energies of X-rays, but in general gamma rays have quantum energies greater than 1 million electron volts ($>1 \times 10^6$ meV), frequencies greater than 1×10^{17} MHz, and wavelengths less than 1×10^{-3} nm.

❍ Are cosmic rays gamma rays from space?

No. Cosmic rays do indeed originate in space, but they are high-energy particles (alpha particles, beta particles, neutrons, or protons) traveling near the speed of light.

❍ What is radioactivity?

The generation of ionizing radiation (which may be particulate or electromagnetic) from atomic nuclei, that is, nuclear radiation.

❍ Is all nuclear radiation ionizing radiation?

Yes.

O   **What are the three most common types of radioactive decay?**

a) Alpha emission (ejection of an alpha particle).

b) Beta emission (ejection of a beta particle [beta particles can be either negatively charged [electrons] or positively charged [positrons]). Three types of beta decay are common in nuclei: Neutron rich nuclei tend to decay by emitting a β- particle. An antineutrino is also emitted in this type of b decay and the it results in the nucleus converting a neutron into a proton. Neutron deficient nuclei tend to decay by positron emission or electron capture. Positron emission refers to the emission of a positron (β+), which is the antiparticle of the electron. A neutrino is emitted in the process and this results in the nucleus converting a proton into a neutron. Electron capture is usually classified as a type of beta decay and involves an orbital electron being absorbed by a nucleus, effectively converting a proton into a neutron.

c) Electron capture (the movement of an electron from the innermost orbit to the nucleus, with the ejection of a neutrino; usually, X-ray radiation from orbital changes by other electrons and gamma rays from the nucleus also occur).

O   **Does gamma-ray emission from the nucleus occur as a sole means of radioactive decay?**

No; although gamma-ray emission may occur in conjunction with alpha emission, beta emission, or electron capture, it never occurs as the sole means of radioactive decay.

O   **What is the difference between a Z number and an A number?**

The Z number refers to the number of protons in an atomic nucleus and is the same as the atomic number of the element; the A number refers to the total number of nucleons (that is, protons and neutrons) in a nucleus.

O   **What are isotopes?**

Forms of an element with the same Z number but different A numbers; that is, they differ only by the number of neutrons in their nuclei.

O   **What is a nuclear decay chain?**

The sequence of events in each step of which an unstable nucleus changes its Z number, its A number, or both, with associated emission of ionizing radiation.

O   **Distinguish between irradiation and induced radiation.**

Irradiation is the exposure of the body to radiation; induced radiation is the induction or creation of radioactivity in an exposed substance or host. In humans, induced radiation is generally produced only by irradiation with neutrons, which may be absorbed by atoms in the body and change them to unstable species that decay via the emission of beta, gamma, and sometimes alpha radiation.

○ **What terms are used to measure activity (radioactivity)?**

Activity (radioactivity), referring to the rate of decay of atomic nuclei, was originally measured by the curie (Ci), representing 3.7 x 1010 disintegrations per second. The new unit in the Système International d'Unités (SI) is the becquerel (Bq), which represents one nuclear decay per second. Thus, 1 Ci = 3.7 x 1010 Bq. Activity measures only the rate of radioactive decay and says nothing about the energy involved in the decay.

○ **How is the amount of non-particulate ionizing radiation (short-wavelength electromagnetic radiation) measured?**

By the roentgen (R). This unit measures the charge produced as X-rays or gamma rays ionize a given volume of air. One roentgen equals 0.000258 coulomb/kilogram (C/kg). Roentgens measure exposure (external dose); to measure intensity, a unit of time must be added, as in roentgens per minute.

○ **Can roentgens be used to measure exposure to corpuscular (particulate) ionizing radiation?**

No.

○ **What do rads and grays measure?**

The absorbed dose either of particulate or of electromagnetic radiation. The rad (radiation absorbed dose) is defined as an absorbed dose of 0.01 joule per kilogram of tissue. The corresponding SI unit, the gray (Gy), represents the dose of any form of radiation resulting in the absorption of 1 joule per kilogram of tissue. Thus, 1 rad = 0.01 Gy. Again, a time unit must be added to change this measure of dose to a measure of intensity, as in Gy/min.

○ **The LD50 (the dose needed to kill 50% of an exposed group) in humans for gamma rays delivered in a short time is about 4 Grays (400 rad). How much thermal energy does this represent?**

9.56 x 10-4 ergs per gram, an amount of thermal energy that would raise the temperature of 1 gram of water less than 0.001° C.

○ **If lethal radiation is so unimpressive expressed as thermal energy, why is it so dangerous?**

The primary effect of thermal energy (as, for example, in microwave and infrared radiation) is to produce molecular vibration. To raise the temperature of a gram of water requires relatively uniform distribution of energy in such a manner that most of the billions of water molecules are induced to vibrate. However, thermal radiation does not have the energy to ionize atoms. Radiation energy, on the other hand, is focused and concentrated to such an extent that if it ejects an electron from a crucial molecule, that ionization can result in the death or mutation of an entire cell.

O   Does 1 rad of particulate radiation cause the same tissue damage as 1 rad of electromagnetic radiation?

Not necessarily; because of the differences in linear energy transfer (LET), particulate radiation is generally more damaging. The "relative biological effectiveness," or RBE, of types of radiation vary. Compared to X-rays and gamma rays, which are defined as having an RBE of 1, high-speed neutrons may have an RBE of 10 to 20 and alpha particles may have an RBE of 20.

O   How is a compensation made for the relative biological effectiveness of different forms of ionizing radiation?

The RBE is used as a "quality factor" (QF) to change the absorbed dose in rads or grays to an equivalent dose.

O   What are the units used to express the biologically effective dose of radiation?

The rem is essentially the dose of any kind of radiation that produces a biological effect equivalent to that from 1 rad of X-rays or gamma rays. Thus, 1 rad of gamma radiation is the same as 1 rem of gamma rays. However, for alpha radiation, which has an RBE, or quality factor, of 20, 1 rad of alpha rays equals 1 rad of gamma radiation times 20, or 20 rem. The applicable SI unit is the sievert (Sv), which represents 100 rem.

O   How does ionizing radiation transfer energy to the body?

By one of three methods:
a) It can transfer all of its energy to an electron as that electron is ejected from the atom. This process is called photoionization (the photoelectric effect), and the ejected electron is called a photoelectron.
b) It can transfer part of its energy to an ejected electron, with the rest becoming a lower-energy (higher-wavelength) photon. This process is called Compton scattering.
c) At very high energies, it can dissociate into an electron-positron pair (pair production). The generated electron and positron then travel through tissue.

O   Describe the penetration and linear-energy-transfer (LET) characteristics of alpha radiation.

Alpha particles, because of their relatively high mass and (except in cosmic rays) relatively slow speed compared to other particulate radiation, they rapidly lose energy over short distances. Their range in air is about 10 cm (4 inches), and they can be stopped by a sheet of paper. They do not penetrate far in tissue. They can pass through a few layers of cells, but alpha particles with energies less than 7.5 MeV cannot completely traverse the 0.07-mm-thick barrier represented by the many layers of keratinized cells in the epidermis. They therefore are not a hazard when present as external radiation on the outside of the body. However, if material containing alpha emitters is inhaled and lodges in the bronchi or bronchioles, the alpha radiation emitted there can damage bronchial epithelium and lead to the development of lung cancer. The high quality factor (Q) of 20 for alpha particles reflects the fact that it has a high LET; that is, as it releases its energy along its relatively short track, the density of ionizations in that region of the cell is very high.

❍ Describe the penetration and linear-energy-transfer (LET) characteristics of beta radiation.

Beta particles have relatively low masses and relatively high speeds. This gives them greater penetrating power than alpha rays. Beta particles differ in energy (speed) depending upon their nuclide of origin; for example, the relatively high-speed beta particles from phosphorus-32 (32P) can travel up to one centimeter in water, whereas the lower-speed beta particles from the decay of tritium (3H) are dissipated after traveling only a tenth of that distance. Beta particles can often travel 3 meters in air and usually penetrate skin to the level of the stratum germinativum, the layer that gives rise to the cells of the rest of the epidermis. They can be blocked by about 3 mm of metal or 6 mm of wood. Their quality factor (Q) is 1, meaning that they have a relatively low linear energy transfer, roughly that of X-rays and gamma rays.

❍ What two types of cellular damage result from ionization of atoms in the body?

a) Direct damage of crucial molecules.
b) Indirect damage mediated by free radicals produced by the ionization of water molecules in the body. The proximate agent in this case is a free radical such as a hyperoxide molecule.

One could also classify the damage as follows:
a) Overt damage (resulting in the death of the involved cell or its inability to undergo mitosis).
b) Occult damage (nonlethal changes in cellular constituents).

Yet another dichotomous classification scheme could be the following:
a) Somatic effects: effects expressed by the affected cell. Somatic effects can be further dichotomized as early (acute) and delayed, or late, effects.
b) Genetic effects: heritable effects caused by alterations in DNA in a cell capable of mitosis.

Still another way of classifying damage would be to use a statistical, population approach:
a) Stochastic effects.
b) Nonstochastic effects.

❍ What is the difference between stochastic and nonstochastic effects?

In nonstochastic processes, the severity but not the frequency of effects rises with increasing dose, but only after the dose passes a given minimal value, or threshold. As the dose of an agent exhibiting a stochastic process increases, the frequency but not severity of effects increases and can be extrapolated back to zero or one (depending upon the scale used). That is, there is no threshold for stochastic events.

❍   **Which radiation effects tend be stochastic in nature, and which tend to be nonstochastic?**

Many of the acute effects of radiation are nonstochastic, but delayed, heritable changes (such as teratogenesis, mutations, and radiation-induced carcinogenesis) appear to be stochastic effects.

❍   **What is ALARA and what does it have to do with stochastic processes?**

Because radiation is presumed to cause certain effects such as cancer via a stochastic process, without a threshold (reflecting the belief that just one single ionization has a low but nonzero chance of leading to cancer) regulations in many countries restrict exposures to radiation to those that are ALARA: As Low As Reasonably Achievable.

❍   **What is the law of Bergonie and Tribondeau (1906)?**

It is the statement that the radiosensitivity of a tissue is directly proportional to its reproductive capacity (in general, its turnover, or mitotic rate) and inversely proportional to its degree of differentiation.

❍   **What is the main exception to the law of Bergonie and Tribondeau?**

Lymphocytes.

❍   **What body tissues are the most exquisitely radiosensitive?**

Lymphocytes.
Immature hematopoietic cells.
Intestinal-crypt cells.
Spermatogonia.
Ovarian follicles.

❍   **List cell types of high to intermediate sensitivity to radiation:**

Most glandular epithelium (breast, bladder, esophagus, stomach).
Oropharyngeal mucous membranes.
Epidermal epithelium.
Endothelium.
Growing bone and cartilage.
Fibroblasts.
Glia.
Epithelium of the lung, kidney, liver, and pancreas.
Thyroid and adrenal glands.

❍   **What body tissues are the least radiosensitive?**

Granulocytes and erythrocytes.

Myocytes.
Mature fibrocytes, bone, and cartilage.
Ganglion cells.

○ **Name several tumors that can arise from exposure to radiation.**

Lymphomas (most forms) and leukemia (lymphocytes and immature hematopoietic cells).
Seminomas and dysgerminomas (spermatogonia).
Granulosa cell tumors (ovarian follicles).
Retinoblastomas (retina).
Transitional cell carcinomas (bladder).
Adenocarcinomas of the stomach.
Carcinomas of the skin, oral cavity, pharynx, esophagus, and cervix.
Small cell carcinomas of the lung.
The vascular (endothelial-cell) and connective-tissue (fibroblastic) components of most tumors.
Osteogenic sarcomas.
Astrocytomas.
Chondrosarcomas.
Bronchogenic (epidermoid) carcinomas of the lung.
Liposarcomas.
Adenocarcinomas of the breast, kidney, thyroid, colon, live, and pancreas.

○ **What radioactive material was responsible for malignant bone tumors in watch-dial painters of the early twentieth century who would lick the tips of their brushes to keep a sharp edge on them?**

Radium.

○ **What radiological contrast agent used in the 1930s and 1940s caused cancer of the liver after its use in diagnostic imaging?**

Thorotrast (thorium dioxide).

○ **What cancers are associated with the highest relative risks in atomic-bomb survivors?**

Leukemia, lymphoma, and cancers of the colon and lung.

○ **What is the average latent period for radiation-induced bone cancers and leukemias?**

About five years, with the risk dropping to near baseline after about two decades.

○ **What is the average latent period for other radiation-induced cancers?**

Ten years or more (in some cases twenty years), with much slower decreases to baseline risk than with bone cancers or leukemias.

○   What is radiation hormesis?

The proposition that low doses of radiation, by stimulating cellular processes of DNA repair, actually reduce the risk of cellular damage associated with radiation. The concept remains intriguing but still controversial.

○   Name several radionuclides (radioactive isotopes) of occupational and environmental concern.

Americium-241 (241Am), cesium-137 (137Cs), cobalt-60 (60Co), radioactive iodine (RAI), phosphorus-32 (32P), plutonium-239 and -238 (239, 238Pu), radium-226 (226Ra), radon-222 (222Rn), strontium-90 (90Sr), tritium (3H), and uranium-238, 235, and 239 (238, 235, 239 U).

○   Describe the use, dangers, and treatment of americium-241 (241Am).

241Am is an alpha emitter found in smoke detectors and other instruments as well as in fallout from nuclear detonations, where it exists as a contaminant with radioactive plutonium. It is also a heavy-metal poison. Diethylenetriaminepentaacetic acid (DTPA, an Investigational New Drug) or calcium edetate (EDTA) are chelators used to remove 241Am from the body.

○   Describe the use, dangers, and treatment of cesium-137 (137Cs).

137Cs, used in medical radiotherapy devices, is both a beta and a gamma emitter. Prussian Blue (an Investigational New Drug for this purpose in the U.S.) and ion-exchange resins are used in treatment.

○   Describe the use, dangers, and treatment of cobalt-60 (60Co).

60Co, which is used both in medical radiotherapy devices and in food irradiators and which might be used in a radiation dispersal device ("dirty bomb"), emits high-energy gamma rays as well as beta radiation. Penicillamine has been suggested as a chelator for severe internal contamination.

○   Describe the use, dangers, and treatment of radioactive iodine (RAI).

Radioactive iodine (RAI) is used to refer to iodine-131, 132, 134, and 135 (131I, 132I, 134I, and 135I), which a normal fission product found in fuel rods of nuclear reactors and which could be released following failure of safety mechanisms at nuclear plants. An example is the Chernobyl release, which resulted in uptake of RAI from the environment and the develop of thyroid cancer especially in children. RAI emits primarily beta rays with some gamma radiation. Potassium iodide (KI) is used to block RAI uptake (see chapter on mass-casualty-weapons I: General, Toxins, and Radiation).

❍ **Describe the use, dangers, and treatment of phosphorus-32 (32P).**

32P, a strong beta emitter, is used as a radioactive tracer in medical facilities and research laboratories. Treatment includes the use of lavage, aluminum hydroxide, and oral phosphates.

❍ **Describe the use, dangers, and treatment of plutonium-239 and plutonium-238 (239Pu and 238Pu).**

239Pu and 238Pu are produced from uranium in reactors and as the primary fissionable material in certain kinds of nuclear weapons is also a chief component of radioactivity from the nuclear or nonnuclear detonation of nuclear weapons. It is always contaminated with americium. Calcium DTPA followed by zinc DTPA is used in chelation of plutonium.

❍ **Describe the use, dangers, and treatment of radium-226 (226Ra).**

226Ra is used for instrument illumination and in industry. An alpha emitter by itself, it is also dangerous because of the alpha, beta, and gamma radiation emitted by its decay products, which include radon-222 (222Rn). (See later questions about radon.) Occupational exposure has been linked to aplastic anemia, leukemia, and osteogenic sarcomas. Ingestion of radium is treated by magnesium sulfate and ammonium chloride.

❍ **Describe the use, dangers, and treatment of strontium-90 (90Sr).**

90Sr, a direct fission product of uranium, emits both beta and gamma radiation, as do its decay products. It tends to follow calcium into bones. Aluminum phosphate given immediately after ingestion can decrease absorption significantly. Nonradioactive strontium can act to compete with 90Sr for uptake into bone. Calcium and acidification of the urine have also been used to increase excretion.

❍ **Describe the use, dangers, and treatment of tritium (3H).**

Tritium, 3H, a beta emitter, is used in various detectors and in nuclear weapons, but because it diffuses quickly into the atmosphere is unlikely to pose a significant radiation hazard. Administration of fluids can accelerate excretion from the body, but overhydration must be avoided.

❍ **Describe the use, dangers, and treatment of uranium-238, uranium-235, and uranium-239 (238U, 235U, and 239U).**

238U, 235U, and 239U are isotopes of increasing radioactivity present (in decreasing abundance) in naturally occurring uranium. They also are present in depleted uranium (in which the proportion of the most radioactive isotopes is reduced) and enriched uranium (in which the proportion of 238U is reduced), used in fuel rods in nuclear weapons and as fissile material in nuclear weapons. These forms of uranium and their decay products emit alpha, beta, and gamma radiation, and if enough enriched uranium is brought together, the resulting critical mass can result in controlled or uncontrolled nuclear fission. Diuresis is used to remove uranyl ion from the body.

○ **What is the average annual human radiation dose from natural and manmade radiation?**

About 300 to 450 mrem.

○ **What proportion of the average annual human radiation dose comes from natural sources?**

About 80%.

○ **On average, what is the largest single source of naturally occurring radiation exposure in humans?**

Radon-222 (222Rn), which is the first decay product of radium 226 (226Ra) (itself a member of the decay series of uranium-238, or 238U) and which represents approximately 55% of the total average annual human radiation dose from all sources.

○ **Can radon by itself directly cause biological damage?**

Yes, by the emission of alpha particles during its transformation to polonium-218 (218Po). However, much of the biological damage caused by radon is caused by alpha, beta, and gamma radiation from decay products of radon.

○ **Give two other terms used to refer to the decay products of radon.**

Radon progeny or radon daughters.

○ **When referring to radon, what is the equilibrium factor?**

The ratio between 222Rn progeny and 222Rn itself. This ratio is typically 0.2 to 0.8, with a mean of about 0.4.

○ **How are radon and its progeny introduced into the body?**

The progeny are adsorbed onto small dust particles suspended in the atmosphere (that is, they form an aerosol), and inhalation of the aerosol results in deposition of the radioactive dust particles in the airways. Decay of radon and radon progeny deposited in the airways generates beta and especially alpha radiation.

○ **Name several occupations at high risk for radon exposure.**

Miners (especially those mining uranium, hard rock, and vanadium).

Other underground workers (e.g., in caves, utility tunnels, radon health mines, subways, underground nuclear-waste repositories, and excavations for construction).
Remediation workers at sites contaminated with radioactivity.
Radon testers and contractors.
Workers in oil refineries, phosphate fertilizer plants, and power plants (especially geothermal and coal plants).
Workers in water plants, fish hatcheries, and radon spas (from waterborne radon).

○   **What are the main sources of radon in buildings?**

Soil and rocks (the most important source of off-gassing), water (including ground water and supplied water, especially from wells), building materials, and outside air.

○   **Does radon exposure cause a particular kind of lung cancer?**

Although early data suggested that radon had a tendency to cause small cell carcinoma of the lung, later data have indicated that the risk is elevated for all types of lung cancer.

○   **When referring to radon, what is a working level (WL)?**

Working level (WL) is a measure of energy released by radon progeny. One working level is any combination of short-lived radon daughters (218Po, 214Pb, 214Bi, and 214Po) that releases 1.3×10^5 MeV of energy from alpha radiation per liter of air. This represents the energy released by the complete decay of these radon daughters in radioactive equilibrium with 222Rn having an activity concentration of 100 picocuries per liter (100 pCi/L). Thus, 1 WL is sometimes equated with 100 pCi/L.

○   **What is a working level month (WLM)?**

A measure of cumulative exposure equivalent to exposure to 1 WL for one working month (170 hours). The corresponding SI unit for cumulative exposure is the joule-hour per cubic meter, or Jh/m3; 1 WLM = 3.5×10^{-3} Jh/m3.

○   **What are the Mine Safety and Health Act (MSHA) and Occupational Safety and Health Act (OSHA) limits for exposure to radon?**

MSHA prohibits employee exposure to more than 1.0 WL (100 pCi/L) in active work areas and limits annual exposure to 4 WLM. OSHA prohibits exposure to more than 0.33 pCi/L or 0.33 WL based upon continuous exposure in the workplace for 40 hours per week and 52 weeks per year (2080 working hours).

○   **What does the Environmental Protection Agency (EPA) recommend as the maximal annual average 222Rn concentration for any occupied area of a home?**

4 pCi/L.

❍   **What types of workers are at the highest risk for radiation exposure?**

Workers at nuclear power plants, other nuclear industrial facilities, or nuclear-powered ships and submarines.
Those working with uranium as fuel for nuclear reactors or components of nuclear weapons.
Workers at storage sites for nuclear waste (including radionuclides from industry and medicine).
Medical technicians and researchers using radionuclides.
Uranium miners and others with exposure to radon and radon daughters (see earlier questions).

❍   **What is the OSHA radiation limit for whole-body general-industry occupational effective radiation dose?**

5 rem (0.05 Sv) per year, or 3 rem (0.03 Sv) in any quarter; this is based on the stochastic risk of cancer and genetic damage.

❍   **What is the OSHA radiation limit for the lens of the eye?**

15 rem (0.15 Sv) per year; this is based on nonstochastic cataract damage.

❍   **What is are the recommendations of the International Commission on Radiological Protection (ICRP) and the National Council on Radiation Protection and Measurements (NCRP) for maximal annual whole-body effective radiation dose for the public?**

0.1 rem (1 mSv). The ICRP allows higher annual doses as long as the annual average over a five-year period does not exceed 0.1 rem. The NCRP allows an annual dose limit of 0.5 rem (5 mSv) when exposure is infrequent as opposed to continuous.

❍   **What types of radiation do film badges measure?**

These badges measure shallow dose and whole-body dose from gamma rays, X-rays, high-energy beta particles, and sometimes neutrons. Low-energy beta radiation, as from tritium (3H), carbon-14 (14C), and sulfur-35 (35S) are unable to penetrate the paper covering the film packet.

❍   **What is a TLD ring?**

A ring, meant to be worn inside a glove with the label facing the palm, which contains a small TLD (thermoluminescent-detector) crystal capable of detecting millicurie amounts of gamma radiation or high-energy beta radiation and of then releasing that energy as light when heated.

❍   **Give examples of local acute effects from radiation exposure.**

Hair loss: beginning at about 300 cGy.
Erythema: above 600 cGy.
Dry desquamation (radionecrosis): above 1,000 cGy.
Wet desquamation: above 2,000 cGy.

❍ **What are the necessary conditions for acquiring acute radiation syndrome (ARS):**

a) The dose must be sufficiently high (usually at least 0.5 to 0.75 Gray).
b) The radiation was able to penetrate the body to reach internal organs.
c) The radiation affects most or all of the body.
d) The radiation is received during a relatively short time interval (usually within minutes).

❍ **What are typically the first clinical signs and symptoms of ARS?**

After a latent period that is inversely correlated with dose and that can range from minutes to days, nausea, vomiting, and diarrhea occur. These are effects of systemic exposure but may also coexist with local effects such as erythema, pruritus, and hair loss. The local effects typically occur after a latent period of several hours.

❍ **What are typical symptoms and signs seen during the prodromal phase of ARS?**

Anorexia, nausea, vomiting, diarrhea, and fatigue with low to moderate doses; with higher doses, fever, difficulty breathing, collapse, and central-nervous-system excitability (including seizures) may also occur.

❍ **What do nausea, vomiting, and diarrhea occurring more than 24 hours after exposure to radiation imply?**

Exposure to a dose less than 0.75 Gray (0.75 Gy).

❍ **How is ARS from doses less than 2 Grays managed?**

By outpatient observation and repeated complete blood counts (CBCs) with differential. Hospitalization is seldom necessary.

❍ **What are the main organ systems systemically affected by high-dose ARS (doses greater than 2 Gy)?**

The hematopoietic system, the gastrointestinal syndrome, the cardiovascular system, and the central nervous system.

❍ **What four distinct phases are usually associated with ARS?**

A prodromal phase of initial symptoms, which may occur shortly after exposure.
A latent phase that may last from minutes to days and is inversely correlated with dose.
An illness phase.
Recovery or death.

❍ **What doses of ionizing radiation are associated with the hematopoietic syndrome?**

Total doses of over 2 Gray (> 2 Gy, or > 200 rad).

○ **Describe the hematopoietic syndrome of ARS.**

Prodromal signs and symptoms may begin within 12 hours with lower doses but within a few hours at higher doses and usually lasts for a day or two. During this time there may be a reactive leukocytosis but a decrease in circulating lymphocytes. During the subsequent symptom-free latent period of up to two to three weeks, absolute lymphocyte counts continue to fall, as do the numbers of neutrophils and platelets. The illness phase is characterized by refractory infections and hemorrhage associated with pancytopenia. Survival of at least some bone marrow irradiated by doses less than 10 Gy is still theoretically possible, and survivors will pass through a recovery period during which hematopoiesis regenerates erythrocytes, leukocytes, and platelets.

○ **What doses of ionizing radiation are associated with the gastrointestinal syndrome?**

Total doses of over 10 Grays (> 10 Gy, or > 1000 rad).

○ **Describe the gastrointestinal syndrome of ARS.**

The prodromal symptoms of nausea, vomiting, and diarrhea occur immediately or very soon after exposure, and the latent period is short. Denudation of gastrointestinal mucosa during the illness phase leads to recurrent nausea and vomiting with bloody diarrhea, dehydration, hemoconcentration, and septicemia. Patients may survive long enough to show elements of the hematopoietic syndrome.

○ **What doses of ionizing radiation are associated with the cardiovascular syndrome?**

Total whole-body doses of over 30 Grays (> 30 Gy, or > 3000 rad).

○ **Describe the cardiovascular/CNS syndrome of ARS.**

Immediate prodromal symptoms of anorexia, nausea, vomiting, and diarrhea may coexist with unstable blood pressure, refractory hypotension, and collapse. The gastrointestinal symptoms may temporarily abate during a latent period never more than a few hours long and followed by central-nervous-system effects such as ataxia, lethargy, loss of consciousness, and convulsions. Death usually occurs within a few days at most. Victims seldom survive long enough to exhibit classic findings of the hematopoietic or gastrointestinal syndromes.

○ **How is ARS managed?**

By observation, supportive care (including comfort measures such as antiemetics), and, in cases where survival is a possibility, attention to the hematopoietic system by means of platelet transfusions, stem-cell transfusions, and the use of growth factors to stimulate hematopoiesis. If exposure has been by means of ingestion, prevention or minimization of cellular uptake of radioactive material is also attempted by using catharsis, gastric lavage, alkalinization of the urine, or administration of heavy-metal chelators such as trisodium zinc diethylenetriaminepentaacetate (Zn-DTPA) or trisodium calcium diethylenetriaminepentaacetate (Ca-DTPA).

❍   **What radioactive elements are considered susceptible to treatment using Zn-DTPA or Ca-DTPA?**

Radioactive rare earths, plutonium, transplutonium elements, and yttrium.

❍   **What radioactive element is considered susceptible to alkalinization of the urine with bicarbonate?**

Uranium.

❍   **What radioactive elements are considered susceptible to treatment using ferric ferrocyanide (Prussian blue)?**

Cesium, rubidium, and thallium.

❍   **What radioactive isotope is considered susceptible to treatment using water?**

Tritium.

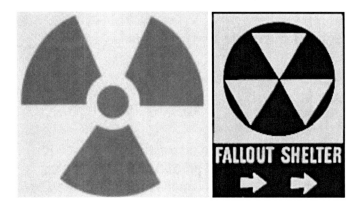

The symbol on the left is the radiation symbol, the most common versions of which use magenta, purple, or black, usually on a yellow background.
The symbol on the right is the symbol for a fallout shelter. Note that it is not the same as the radiation symbol.

OCCUPATIONALLY RELATED INFECTIOUS DISEASES

○ **What general types of organisms cause disease in workers?**

Viruses, rickettsiae, chlamydiae, bacteria, fungi, and parasites.

○ **What term is preferred to infection to describe a condition caused by a parasite?**

Infestation.

○ **Compare rickettsiae and chlamydiae to viruses and bacteria.**

Like viruses, both rickettsiae and chlamydiae are both obligate intracellular parasites; like bacteria, their metabolism is independent of host cellular activity and they are susceptible to antibiotics.

○ **Structurally, what distinguishes Gram-negative bacteria from Gram-positive bacteria?**

The presence in Gram-negative bacteria of a toxic lipopolysaccharide cell-wall component.

○ **What is the name given to the toxic lipopolysaccharide in Gram-negative bacteria?**

Endotoxin.

○ **What are Koch's postulates?**

The organism thought to be causative for the disease must be found in naturally diseased but not healthy animals.
The suspected organisms must be isolated from the diseased animal and grown in pure culture.
Inoculation of healthy animals by a pure culture of the suspected organism must produce the same disease seen in naturally occurring cases.
Organisms isolated by culture of inoculated diseased animals must be indistinguishable from organism isolated from animals with naturally occurring disease.

○ **By what routes are infectious diseases transmitted in humans?**

Inhalation, or respiratory, transmission (including inhalation of airborne droplets).
Oral, or enteral, transmission (including ingestion of airborne droplets).
Direct contact.
Parenteral transmission.

Transmission via arthropod vectors.

Another, albeit somewhat more ambiguous, way of classifying modes of transmission is the following:
  a) Direct.
  b) Indirect.
  c) Airborne (sometimes listed independently, and sometimes listed as a subset of indirect transmission).

The following classification scheme is used by the Centers for Disease Control and Prevention (CDC):
  a) Contact transmission.
      1) Direct-contact transmission (direct body contact).
      2) Indirect-contact transmission (contact via fomites).
  b) Droplet transmission.
  c) Airborne transmission.
  d) Common-vehicle transmission (via, e.g., food, water, medications, devices, and equipment).
  e) Vectorborne transmission (via arthropods or other small living organisms).

❍ **Distinguish between droplet transmission and airborne transmission.**

Droplet transmission, theoretically a form of contact transmission, involves transmission by means of relatively large droplets produced during coughing, sneezing, talking, and certain medical procedures. These particles typically do not travel more than a few feet in air before settling. Airborne transmission refers to transmission by much smaller droplet nuclei, 5 microns or less in aerodynamic diameter. These nuclei remain suspended in air for much longer periods of time than do the larger droplets involved in droplet transmission.

❍ **What are the four kinds of precautions currently recommended by the Centers for Disease Prevention and Control (CDC) for infection control?**

Standard precautions.
Airborne precautions.
Droplet precautions.
Contact precautions.

❍ **Elements of what two former kinds of precautions were combined to generate standard precautions?**

a) Universal precautions, or UP (for bloodborne pathogens); and b) body substance isolation, or BSI (for moist and potentially infective body surfaces).

❍ **Describe standard precautions.**

Standard precautions are designed to reduce the risk of transmission of bloodborne pathogens of pathogens from moist body substances and apply to a) blood; b) all bodily fluids, secretions, and excretions except sweat; c) nonintact skin; and d) mucous membranes and include a variety of protective measures, including handwashing, gloving, masking, gowning, prevention of needlestick injuries, adequate disinfection, and the use of private rooms as appropriate.

○ **Describe airborne precautions.**

Airborne precautions include, in addition to the measures indicated for standard precautions, patient placement in a private room with a closed door, monitored negative air pressure relative to the surrounding area, six to 12 air changes per hour, and appropriate processing and discharge of air; adequate respiratory protection; and limitation of patient transport.

○ **Describe droplet precautions.**

Droplet precautions require patient placement in a private room, masking when within three feet of the patient, and limitation of patient transport in addition to standard precautions.

○ **Describe contact precautions.**

Contact precautions supplement standard precautions with special procedures (relating especially to gowning, masking, and processing of equipment coming in contact with the patient) designed to minimize the risk of transmission of infectious organisms present on the patient's skin.

○ **Contrast reservoir with vector and host.**

A reservoir is the environmental source or the infectious agent of a disease and can be man, arthropod species, other animal species, species of plant, soil, or other environmental substance where the infectious agents normally lives and reproduces. Vectors are living organisms (usually insects or other arthropods) that transmit an infectious agent from its reservoir to its host. A host is the organism whose disease is the one under consideration. Hosts, vectors, and reservoirs may overlap depending upon the perspective.

○ **Distinguish colonization from infection.**

Colonization refers to the presence of microorganisms in a healthy host; infection refers to presence both of organisms and also of disease produced by the microorganisms.

○ **Define endemic, pandemic, and epidemic.**

Endemic refers to a disease that exists stably or constantly within a given reservoir or area. Disease seen in an extremely large area or reservoir is said to be pandemic, whereas epidemic refers to the occurrence of disease in a sharply elevated rate in a given community.

○ **Define zoonosis, enzootic, and epizootic.**

A zoonosis is an infectious disease transmitted under natural conditions from vertebrate animals to humans. Enzootic and epizootic correspond in animal populations to endemic and epidemic, respectively, in human populations.

○   **There are over 200 zoonoses. Name three occupationally important zoonoses.**

Brucellosis.
Leptospirosis.
Orf.
Psittacosis.
Q fever.
[many others are possible]

○   **What is an arbovirus?**

A virus typically transmitted by an arthropod vector.

○   **What represents the illness most frequently associated with absence from work?**

The common cold (upper respiratory infections caused by rotaviruses, coronaviruses, and other viruses).

○   **Is the common cold usually considered to be an occupationally related infectious disease? Why or why not?**

Occupationally related infectious diseases usually refer to those diseases with higher rates among a specific occupational group than in the community at large. Since the rate of infection with the common cold does not differ substantially between the work environment and the general environment, the common cold would not normally be considered to be occupationally related even though its incidence in the workplace is appreciable.

○   **What bloodborne viruses are particularly relevant to healthcare workers?**

Hepatitis B virus (HBV), hepatitis C virus (HCV), and human immunodeficiency virus (HIV).

○   **What are the estimated risks of acquiring infection from hepatitis B virus (HBV), hepatitis C virus (HCV) and human immunodeficiency-virus (HIV) from a single needlestick?**

Approximately 30% for HBV, 3% for HCV, and 0.3% for HIV.

○   **According to the U.S. Public Health Service (USPHS), what are the four major factors to consider in assessing the need for follow-up of occupational exposures to HBV, HBC, HCV, and HIV?**

a) Type of exposure:

Percutaneous injury.
Exposure to mucous membranes.
Exposure to nonintact skin.
Bites resulting in blood exposure to either person involved.

b) Type and amount of fluid/tissue:
Blood.
Fluids containing blood.
Potentially infectious fluid or tissue (semen; vaginal secretions; and cerebrospinal, synovial, pleural, peritoneal, pericardial, and amniotic fluids).
Direct contact with concentrated virus.

c) Infectious state of source:
Presence of HBsAg.
Presence of HCV antibody.
Presence of HIV antibody.

d) Susceptibility of exposed person.
Hepatitis B vaccine and vaccine response status.
HBC, HCV, and HIV immune status.

O   **What does the presence of hepatitis B surface antigen (HBsAg) in a worker denote?**

The presence of infectious virus.

O   **What does the presence of antibodies to HBsAg (anti-HBs) in a worker denote?**

Past infection, immune response to HBV vaccine, or presence of hepatitis B immune globulin (HBIG).

O   **About what proportion of American adults infected with HBV are carriers?**

About 5-10%.

O   **What are the long-term sequelae of infection with HBV?**

Chronic active hepatitis.
Cirrhosis.
Primary hepatocellular carcinoma. (Liver CA)

O   **What does the USPHS recommend for post-exposure prophylaxis (PEP) of HBV-vaccinated healthcare workers percutaneously exposed to an HBsAg-positive source?**

It depends upon the responder status of the healthcare worker. Known responders need no treatment, known responders are given either one dose of HBIG and revaccination or else two doses of HBIG. Those whose responder status is unknown are tested for anti-HBs and then treated according to the response status indicated by the test.

O   **Infection with hepatitis C virus (HCV) accounts for about what proportion of infections initially designated non-A, non-B (NANB) hepatitis?**

Approximately 90%.

O   **Approximately what percentage of HCV-infected individuals become chronic carriers, with persistent viremia?**

About 80%.

O   **Approximately what percentage of HCV-infected individuals go on to develop end-stage liver disease?**

About 20 to 25%.

O   **Does HCV infection raise the risk for the development of hepatocellular carcinoma?**

Yes; about one third of the cases of hepatocellular carcinoma (HCC) in the U.S. occur in HCV-positive individuals, although almost all of the HCC cases in HCV-positive individuals occur in those who have first developed cirrhosis or advanced fibrosis.

O   **What is the currently recommended antiviral postexposure prophylaxis for healthcare workers percutaneously exposed to blood from an HCV-positive individual?**

No antiviral agents are currently recommended for postexposure prophylaxis after exposure to HCV-positive blood.

O   **About what percentage of individuals who become positive for human immunodeficiency virus (HIV) develop acquired immune deficiency syndrome (AIDS) within ten years of seroconversion?**

About 54%.

O   **What are the three main classes of antiretroviral agents?**

(a) Nucleoside reverse transcriptase inhibitors (NRTIs):
       Zidovudine (ZDV; AZT; Retrovir™).
       Lamivudine (3TC; Epivir™).
       Stavudine (d4T; Zerit™).
       Didanosine (DDI; Videx™).
       Abacavir (ABC; Ziagen™).

(b) Nonnucleoside reverse transcriptase inhibitors (NNRTIs):

Nevirapine (NVP; Viramune™).
Delavirdine (DLV; Rescriptor™).
Efavirenz (EFV; Sustiva™).

c) Protease inhibitors (PIs):
Indinavir (IDV; Crixivan™).
Nelfinavir (NFV; Viracept™).
Ritonavir (RTV; Norvir™).
Saquinavir (SQV; Fortovase™).
Amprenavir (AMP; Agenerase™).
Lopinavir/Ritonavir (Kaletra™).

○ **With reference to HIV postexposure prophylaxis (PEP), what are the two categories of HIV-positive patients?**

a) HIV-positive Class I patients: Asymptomatic patients or patients with a viral load known to be low (e.g., < 1,500 RNA copies/mL).
b) HIV-positive Class II patients:
Symptomatic HIV patients.
AIDS patients.
Patients with acute seroconversion.
Patients with a viral load known to be high (e.g., > 1,500 RNA copies/mL).

○ **With reference to HIV PEP, what are the two relevant types of percutaneous HIV exposure?**

Less severe exposures, e.g., injuries from solid needles and superficial injuries.
More severe exposures, e.g., large-bore hollow-needle injuries, deep puncture wounds, visible blood on the device, or injury from a needle used in an artery or vein of a patient.

○ **With reference to HIV PEP, what are the two relevant types of exposures to mucous membranes or nonintact skin?**

Small-volume exposures, e.g., a few drops.
Large-volume exposures, e.g., a large splash.

○ **What are the U.S. Public Health Service (USPHS) recommendations for PEP for less severe percutaneous exposures?**

Basic 2-drug PEP if the source is HIV-positive Class I.
Expanded 3-drug PEP if the source is HIV-positive Class II.
No PEP if the source HIV status is unknown but risk factors are low.
Basic 2-drug PEP if source HIV status is unknown but risk factors are high.
No PEP if the source is unknown but the exposure setting is low-risk.
Basic 2-drug PEP if the source is unknown but exposure to HIV-positive persons is likely.
No PEP if the source is HIV-negative.

○   **What are the U.S. Public Health Service (USPHS) recommendations for PEP for more severe percutaneous exposures?**

The recommendations are identical to those for less severe exposures with the exception that for more severe exposures expanded 3-drug PEP is recommended if the source is HIV-positive Class I.

○   **What are the U.S. Public Health Service (USPHS) recommendations for PEP for small-volume exposures to mucous membranes or to nonintact skin?**

Basic 2-drug PEP if the source is HIV-positive Class I (strategy offered for consideration).
Basic 2-drug PEP if the source is HIV-positive Class II.
No PEP if the source HIV status is unknown but risk factors are low.
Basic 2-drug PEP if source HIV status is unknown but risk factors are high.
No PEP if the source is unknown but the exposure setting is low-risk.
Basic 2-drug PEP if the source is unknown but exposure to HIV-positive persons is likely.
No PEP if the source is HIV-negative.

○   **What are the U.S. Public Health Service (USPHS) recommendations for PEP for large-volume exposures to mucous membranes or to nonintact skin?**

The recommendations are identical to those for small-volume exposures except that a) basic 2-drug PEP for Class I HIV-positive sources is recommended rather than simply offered for consideration and b) expanded 3-drug PEP is recommended if the source is HIV-positive Class II.

○   **How does the risk of infection with cytomegalovirus (CMV) in healthcare workers compare with the risk of CMV infection in the general population?**

They are about the same.

○   **What viral disease caused by a paramyxovirus affects the eyes of poultry handlers, laboratory workers, and veterinarians?**

Newcastle disease.

○   **A poxvirus found especially in sheep and goats but also occasionally in deer and reindeer can cause either a solitary red to violet skin lesion or (less commonly) multiple skin lesions. The initial lesion can begin as a papule, vesicle, or nodule but usually develops central umbilication with serous drainage. It may also become secondarily infected. Occasionally, a maculopapular truncal rash accompanies the skin lesion or lesions. The infection can be spread to the eyes and may become disseminated. Erythema multiforme is a reported complication. What is the disease?**

Human orf, also called orf virus disease and echthyma contagiosum.

○   **What are the causative agents of louseborne typhus fever and fleaborne typhus fever?**

All forms of typhus fever are rickettsial in origin. Rickettsia prowazekii is responsible for epidemic louseborne typhus fever (classic typhus fever) and R. typhi (R. mooseri) and R. felis cause endemic fleaborne typhus fever (murine typhus, or shop typhus), which is transmitted by rodents carrying flea vectors. Another form of typhus, scrub typhus, or miteborne typhus fever, is caused by Orienta tsutsugamushi (Rickettsia tsutsugamushi).

○   **Name a rickettsial disease that affects the liver, the lung, and the brain and that poses a risk to slaughterhouse (abattoir) workers, farmers, ranchers, and laboratory workers by means of contact with placental tissue, urine, or stool from infected cattle, sheep, goats, and wild animals.**

Q fever, (caused by Coxiella burnetii.)   *tick*

○   **Name a rickettsial disease that is spread by ticks from infected rodents and dogs and that constitutes a risk for forest workers, ranchers, farmers, and hunters.**

Rocky Mountain spotted fever (RMSF), (caused by Rickettsia rickettsii.)

○   **What is the causative agent of ornithosis, what occupational groups are at risk, and what are the usual vehicles of transmission?**

Ornithosis, caused by the chlamydial organism Chlamydia psittaci, is a risk for zoo attendants, poultry workers, pet-shop employees, and other bird handlers who contact urine, stool, or other discharges (or inhale chlamydia-containing dust) from infected pigeons or domestic birds such as parrots and parakeets.

○   **What workers are at the greatest risk for developing anthrax?**

Workers dealing with animal hides, hair, bone, and wool (including weavers); veterinarians; and wildlife workers.

○   **What is the causative organism of anthrax?**

Bacillus anthracis, a spore-forming, (Gram-positive, rod-shaped bacterium.)

○   **What is the most common occupationally related form of anthrax?**

Cutaneous anthrax ("wool-sorters' disease"), characterized by painless black ulcers that progress to necrotic eschars. Anthrax also occurs in other forms and is a CDC Category A biological agent (see chapter on mass-casualty weapons II: biological agents).

○   **What workers are at the greatest risk of acquiring brucellosis?**

Slaughterhouse (abattoir) workers, farmers, dairy workers, and veterinarians.

○ **What are the causative agents of brucellosis?**

Brucellosis abortus, B. melitensis, B. suis, and B. canis, all of which are gram-negative coccobacillary bacteria found in contaminated milk products (B. abortus), goats (B. melitensis), sheep (B. melitensis), swine (B. suis), and dogs (B. canis). They can be transmitted through ingestion, inhalation, and skin contact.

○ **What are the clinical features of brucellosis?**

The disease may have either an acute or a gradual onset, with variable fever ("undulant fever") and chills, headache, myalgias, arthralgias, lymphadenopathy, chronic hepatitis, genitourinary infections, and a high incidence of complications involving joint inflammation. Brucellosis is also a CDC Category B biological agent.

○ **A relatively recently described tick-borne disease in the U.S. causes nonspecific symptoms (malaise, fever, headache, nausea, vomiting, anorexia, and myalgia) that may progress to a fatal outcome. Outdoor workers are at risk. The disease is caused by bacteria that were once classified in the genus Rickettsia. What is the disease, and what organisms cause it?**

Ehrlichiosis has two major forms: Human mononuclear ehrlichiosis (HME) primarily affects monocytes and is caused by Ehrlichia chaffeensis, and human granulocytic ehrlichiosis (HGE) is caused by E. phagocytophila, E. equi, or related species. These bacteria are currently classified in the tribe Ehrlichieae of the family Rickettsiaceae.

○ **What is the causative organism of erysipeloid, and what workers are at risk of this disease?**

Erysipeloid, caused by Erysipelothrix rhusiopathiae (insidiosa), is a skin disease contracted by fishermen, fish processors, meat and poultry workers, and veterinarians exposed to infected shellfish, fish, meat, and poultry. However, this Gram-positive filamentous bacterium can also cause septicemia and endocarditis.

○ **What organ systems does leptospirosis affect, what workers are at risk, and how is the disease acquired?**

Leptospirosis, which is caused by the spirochetal bacterium Leptospira interrogans and which affects the liver, the kidney, and the brain, is also known as Weil disease, Canicola fever, or hemorrhagic jaundice. Field workers (including sugarcane and rice harvesters), slaughterhouse (abattoir) workers, farmers, sewer workers, veterinarians, miners, and fishermen are among workers at risk. The disease can be spread either by contaminated water or by tissue, urine, or feces of infected rodents or other animals (wild or domesticated).

О **Outdoor workers are at increased risk of developing Lyme disease. What is the causative agent of Lyme disease?**

The spirochete Borrelia burgdorferi.

О **What is the main species that serves as a vector for Lyme disease?**

The tick species Ixodes. Ixodes scapularis, the black-legged tick, is the main vector in the southeastern U.S. Ixodes dammini, the Northern deer tick, is the principal vector in the Northeast but is not universally accepted as a species distinct from I. scapularis. The main vector in the western U.S. is I. pacificus, the Western black-legged tick.

О **What are the three stages in the development of the ticks that transmit Lyme disease?**

Larvae, nymphs, and adults.

О **On what animals do the ticks that transmit Lyme disease feed?**

Larvae and nymphs can feed on many mammals, birds, and reptiles but prefer Peromyscus leucopus, the white-footed mouse. Adults feed primarily on Odocoileus virginianus, the white-tailed deer. Each stage feeds only once.

О **Which stage of tick is responsible for most human cases of Lyme disease?**

The nymph stage.

О **How long is it thought that ticks need to feed on their hosts before becoming capable of infecting humans with Borrelia burgdorferi?**

24 to 48 hours.

О **Describe the early clinical presentation (localized early infection) of Lyme disease.**

Initial symptoms and signs may include fatigue, malaise, and fever and are accompanied in 60% to 90% of cases by one or more expanding annular erythematous macules (often with central clearing) referred to as erythema migrans (EM). However, EM-like lesions can be seen in a variety of conditions, and the absence of EM does not exclude Lyme disease. This stage was originally designated Stage I disease.

О **Describe the next stage (disseminated early infection) of Lyme disease.**

Systemic involvement is often heralded within days or weeks by myalgias and migratory arthralgias. In 10% to 20% of cases in the U.S., headache and stiff neck may indicate involvement of the central nervous system (CNS). Other CNS manifestations may include cranial neuropathy (e.g., Bell's palsy), peripheral neuropathy, radiculitis, myelitis, and meningitis. In 4% to 10% of cases, cardiac involvement is seen as myocarditis and a variety of dysrhythmias. Dissemination to the eye can lead to conjunctivitis and keratitis. These signs and symptoms may last weeks to months and may be constant or intermittent. This stage was formerly known as Stage II Lyme disease.

O **Describe the clinical manifestations of persistent, or late, Lyme disease.**

This stage, originally called Stage III Lyme disease, may be seen either as persistent or recurrent disease within months to years of the initial infection and lasting for months to year. Arthritis may occur as months-long episodes or as persistent chronic disease. Memory loss and subtle behavioral changes may occur, as may a progressive encephalomyelitis with frank dementia, ataxia, and involvement of cranial and peripheral nerves.

O **What antibiotics are most frequently recommended for postexposure prophylaxis and treatment of those exposed to Lyme disease?**

Doxycycline, amoxicillin, and erythromycin.

O **Yersinia pestis is the Gram-negative coccobacillary bacterium that causes plague. In what occupational settings does bubonic plague usually occur?**

Veterinarians, zookeepers, and laboratory workers who come in contact with infected animals or with fleas from infected animals may acquire bubonic disease from the bites of infected fleas. However, hunters and trappers may develop this form of plague from direct transmission of the plague bacillus into abraded or otherwise nonintact skin during skinning. Plague is also a CDC Category A biological agent (see the chapter on mass-casualty weapons II: biological agents).

O **Listeria monocytogenes, a Gram-positive, rod-shaped bacterium, causes listeriosis, which may lead to sepsis with involvement of brain and meninges. Veterinarians are at increased risk. In what other occupational groups is the risk for listeriosis increased?**

Veterinarians are the only workers documented to have an increased risk of contracting listeriosis.

O **Pig farmers, meat packers, and butchers exposed to raw pork via cuts or minor breaks in the skin (and possibly by inhalation of infective material as well) may develop a flu-like syndrome with sepsis, meningeal involvement, and a characteristic early-onset hearing loss that may become permanent. What organism is responsible for this disease?**

Streptococcus suis Type II, a Group R beta-hemolytic streptococcus.

O **Construction workers, gardeners, farmers, and others who work in close contact with soil are at risk for tetanus, which is caused by Clostridium tetani. How does the paralysis produced by C. tetani differ from the paralysis produced by C. botulinum?**

Clostridium tetani produces a rigid, tetanic paralysis as opposed to the flaccid paralysis caused by C. botulinum.

○ **What workers are at the greatest risk of developing tuberculosis?**

Healthcare workers (especially those dealing with respiratory infections and performing invasive procedures on patients with respiratory conditions), prison workers, homeless-shelter workers, drug-treatment workers, pathologists, morticians, and workers with silicosis. Workers who are otherwise at risk for tuberculosis because of poor socioeconomic status or association with groups having high incidences of the disease are also at risk, but not necessarily because of their specific kind of employment.

○ **What categories of individuals are considered to be at such a high risk of developing tuberculosis that their screening purified-protein-derivative (PPD, or Mantoux) skin test is considered positive if there is any reaction greater than 5 mm in diameter?**

HIV-infected individuals.
Close recent contacts of an active case of tuberculosis.
Individuals with a chest radiograph consistent with old tuberculosis.

○ **What categories of individuals are considered to be at such a high risk of developing tuberculosis that their screening purified-protein-derivative (PPD, or Mantoux) skin tests are considered positive is there is any reaction greater than 5 mm in diameter?**

HIV-infected individuals.
Close recent contacts of an active case of tuberculosis.
Individuals with a chest radiograph consistent with old tuberculosis.

○ **What categories of individuals are considered to be at an intermediate risk of developing tuberculosis, such that their screening purified-protein-derivative (PPD, or Mantoux) skin tests are considered positive if there is any reaction greater than 10 mm in diameter?**

Foreign-born individuals.
Users of intravenous drugs.
Residents of long-term-care institutions.
Low-income groups.
High-risk racial or ethnic minorities.
Those with certain medical conditions, such as gastrectomy, diabetes mellitus, and immune-system compromise.

○ **In those individuals considered to be at low risk for the development of tuberculosis, what is the minimal diameter of the reaction to a PPD (Mantoux) skin test for the test to be considered to be positive?**

15 mm.

○ **What is the prime characteristic used to grade the response to a PPD (Mantoux) skin test?**

Induration (not erythema).

○ **What is the causative organism of tuberculosis?**

Mycobacterium tuberculosis, a slowly growing acid-fast mycobacterium (a true bacterium that resembles a fungus in some ways).

○ **Distinguish between tuberculosis infection and tuberculosis disease.**

Tuberculosis infection is a term widely used to refer to the presence of tuberculosis bacteria in tissues without overt clinical indications of disease, although the more technically correct term in this case would be tuberculosis colonization. Tuberculosis disease, or active tuberculosis, refers to pathological changes manifesting themselves in clinical symptoms or signs. Tuberculosis infection is not considered to be transmissible; tuberculosis disease is transmissible.

○ **How is tuberculosis disease transmitted?**

Tuberculosis is transmitted by airborne droplet nuclei less than 5 mm in diameter. These droplets can remain suspended in the air for significant periods of time. Patients with cavitary disease, cough of long duration, copious and watery sputum, and large numbers of acid-fast bacteria in their sputum are particularly infectious. However, less than a third of close contacts of those with tuberculosis disease become infected.

○ **About what percentage of individuals infected with tuberculosis go on to develop clinical disease?**

About 10%.

○ **About what percentage of HIV-infected individuals who become infected with tuberculosis go on to develop clinical tuberculosis?**

About 60 to 80%.

○ **In addition to airborne precautions (including negative-pressure ventilation with at least six air exchanges per hour), what else does the Advisory Council for the Elimination of Tuberculosis (ACET) recommend be done with air from rooms with patients who have tuberculosis disease?**

The air should undergo ultraviolet radiation to kill tuberculosis bacteria.

○ **What is the minimal efficiency required of a respirator to protect against tuberculosis?**

95% efficiency; that is, an N95 mask is the minimal requirement. Surgical masks worn either by a tuberculosis patient or a healthcare provider may protect the tuberculosis patient against infections transmitted by others but do not protect healthcare workers from becoming infected with tuberculosis.

O **What workers are at the greatest risk of acquiring infection with other mycobacterial organisms?**

Healthcare workers may acquire infection with Mycobacterium kansasii or M. avium intracellulare from hospital patients. Dairy-cattle workers can become infected with M. bovis, and fish infected with M. marinum can transmit this organism via skin contact to workers who handle fish.

O **What occupational groups are most at risk for contracting tularemia?**

Tularemia, caused by the small coccobacillary Gram-negative bacterium Francisella tularensis, has skin and systemic forms and can be transmitted to hunters, farmers, forest workers, trappers, veterinarians, and laboratory workers via bites from infected animals or arthropods, ingestion of contaminated meat, or contact with or inhalation of dust or other material contaminated by blood, urine, or other secretions from infected animals. Tularemia is also a CDC Category A biological agent (see the chapter on mass-casualty weapons II: biological agents).

O **Name important fungal diseases of occupational relevance in the U.S. and their causative organisms.**

(desert or Valley Fever)

Blastomycosis (Blastocystis dermatitidis) , coccidioidomycosis (Coccidioides immitis), histoplasmosis (Histoplasma capsulatum), and sporotrichosis (Sporothrix schenckii).

O **Describe the sources, routes of exposure, and workers at risk for blastomycosis.**

Blastocystis organisms are found in soil (in the U.S., predominantly in the Midwest and in the Southeast) and in dogs and can enter the body by being inhaled or ingested or through a dog bite. Workers most at risk are those whose work puts them into direct contact with soil; thus, farmers, plant-nursery workers, horticulturists, and construction workers are among high-risk groups.

O **Describe the clinical manifestations of blastomycosis.**

Blastomycosis affects the lungs (causing both acute and also chronic pneumonia), the skin (where it may give rise to wart-like lesions, ulcers, and subcutaneous nodules), and bone (where it may cause a chronic osteomyelitis with bone resorption and draining sinuses).

O **Describe the sources, routes of exposure, and workers at risk for coccidioidomycosis.**

Coccidioides immitis exists in soil (including land fills) in dry regions of the American Southwest (from California to Texas), cotton, and fruit. Infection is usually by inhalation of dust containing C. immitis. Workers at risk include outdoor workers such as archaeologists, migrant workers, and military personnel who work in or travel through endemic areas, especially in summers following a rainy spring. Healthcare workers exposed to infective spores from, for examples, moist casts, can also acquire the disease.

O   **Describe the clinical presentation of coccidioidomycosis.**

Coccidioidomycosis, also called desert fever or valley fever, has an acute phase that typically involves the lungs. Cavitation and pulmonary nodules may develop, and patients may also develop the skin lesions of erythema nodosum. In the estimated 0.1% of cases that lead to systemic infection, nodules and abscesses may develop not only in the lungs but also in and under the skin, in bone, and in the meninges. Systemic disease is not uncommonly fatal.

O   **Describe the sources, routes of exposure, and workers at risk for histoplasmosis.**

Histoplasma capsulatum frequents soil contaminated with feces from birds (particularly pigeons, starlings, and blackbirds) and bats. Construction workers (including soil movers), pigeon and chicken handlers, street cleaners, spelunkers, and archaeologists could be expected to acquire the fungus by inhalation.

O   **Describe the clinical presentation of histoplasmosis.**

The main form, American histoplasmosis, exists in several forms, including an asymptomatic variant, mild respiratory symptoms, an acute disseminated form (which spreads to affect the liver, the spleen, lymph nodes, and bone marrow and if usually fatal if untreated), chronic systemic disease, and chronic pulmonary histoplasmosis, which with its cavitary lesions resembles tuberculosis radiographically. The less common skin variant of histoplasmosis has been described only in Africa and Madagascar.

O   **Describe the sources, routes of exposure, and workers at risk for sporotrichosis.**

The fungus responsible for sporotrichosis resides in soil and plants and is typically acquired by inoculation through the skin in plant handlers (for example, from scratches by rose thorns or by handling sphagnum moss), lumber workers (from splinters), and miners. Less commonly, organisms can be inhaled.

O   **Summarize the clinical features of sporotrichosis.**

A skin nodule at the site of exposure may soften and ulcerate and may precede the development of similar nodules along draining lymphatic channels, which themselves may become hard and rope-like. Disseminated disease is possible but uncommon.

O   **With reference to parasitism, define reservoir host, intermediate host, and definitive host.**

A reservoir host is an organism in or on which a parasite lives in nature. An intermediate host is an organism in which the larval or asexual stage of a parasite is found. A definitive host is an organism in which a parasite undergoes sexual reproduction. Definitive hosts can also be reservoir hosts, or reservoirs, for parasites.

❍ **With reference to parasitism, what is the difference between a biological vector and a mechanical vector?**

Both are animals (usually arthropods) that are capable of transmitting a parasite, but a biological vector is essential for parasite development or reproduction, whereas a mechanical vector simply transfers a parasite from one organism to another without being a necessary part of the life cycle of the parasite.

❍ **Parasites include one-celled protozoans and also helminths (worms). Describe the different types of parasitic helminths.**

Annelids, such as leeches, are segmented worms. Nematodes are roundworms; parasitic roundworms are also called ascarids. Platyhelminths, or flatworms, include trematodes (flukes) and cestodes (tapeworms).

❍ **In terms of the parasites involved, what is the difference between toxoplasmosis and toxocariasis?**

Toxoplasmosis is caused by the intracellular coccidian protozoan Toxoplasma gondii, which infests the intestinal epithelium of cats. Intermediate hosts include herbivores, rodents, and birds. Toxocariasis, also known as visceral larval migrans, is caused by the ascarid nematodes Toxocara canis and Toxocara cati, which infest dogs and cats, respectively. Those who work with cats and dogs are therefore at risk of developing toxocariasis.

❍ **Humans serve as reservoirs for which two species of hookworms?**

Necator americanus and Ancylostoma duodenale.

❍ **How do hookworms usually enter the body, and what occupational groups are at risk?**

Hookworm larvae penetrate the skin of unprotected feet in farmers, excavators, sewer workers, and recreation workers who work in contaminated water. The larvae then travel via blood vessels or lymphatics to the lungs, migrate from the alveoli and airways to the pharynx, are swallowed, and eventually attach themselves to intestinal epithelium.

❍ **Describe the agents, the workers at risk, and the sources of infection for echinococcosis.**

Echinococcosis, caused by the larval forms of the tapeworms Echinococcus granulosis and Echinococcus multilocularis, results from the ingestion of tapeworm eggs in the feces of infected dogs, foxes, or related animals. Ingestion can be from hand-to-mouth transmission after direct contact with the animals or their feces or from fomites. Veterinarians, ranchers, sheepherders, and others in close occupational contact with dogs are at risk, as are children.

○   What are the definitive hosts and intermediate hosts for Echinococcus granulosis?

The principal definitive host for Echinococcus granulosis is the domestic dog, although the tapeworm can also undergo sexual reproduction in foxes and other canids. Cats and other felines do not serve as hosts for this parasite. Intermediate hosts include herbivores such as sheep, cattle, goats, pigs, and horses.

○   What are the definitive hosts and intermediate hosts for Echinococcus multilocularis?

Although dogs and cats can serve as definitive hosts for Echinococcus multilocularis, the principal definitive hosts are wild animals such as foxes. Wild rodents act as intermediate hosts.

○   Echinococcosis can also be caused by Echinococcus vogeli. Why is this not considered an occupational disease in the U.S.?

Because it is primarily found in Latin America.

○   How do echinococcal tapeworms lead to human disease?

Ingested eggs release infective embryos, or oncospheres, which are delivered by the blood to the lung, the liver, the brain, and other organs, where they form fluid-filled, or hydatid, cysts.

○   Define emerging infectious disease (EID).

An emerging infectious disease is one which has become more prevalent in humans during the past twenty years or is thought likely to become more prevalent in the near future.

○   List at three diseases considered to be emerging infectious diseases in the U.S.

Coccidioidomycosis.
Cryptosporidiosis.
Drug-resistant pneumococcal disease.
Infection with Escherichia coli O157:H7.
Hantavirus pulmonary syndrome (HPS).
Vancomycin-resistant enterococcal infections.

WORKERS' COMPENSATION

○ **What are the top five work related causes of death reported for compensation to Workers' Compensation?**

Motor vehicle accidents, falls, electric shock, burns and non-ingested poisonings.

○ **What is the most common disabling injury reported to Workers' Compensation?**

Overexertion.

○ **What is the most commonly injured body part reported to Workers' Compensation?**

The back.

○ **What is the second most commonly injured body part reported?**

The legs.

○ **Prior to Workers' Compensation laws, what must an employee prove to get compensated for injury?**

That the employer was responsible for injury or death resulting from the employers negligence.

○ **What doctrine was successfully used by employers to counter claims of liability prior to workman's compensation laws?**

Contributory negligence on the part of the employee, fellow employee negligence, and assumed risk of the job for payment.

○ **Who must prove fault under the Workers' Compensation laws?**

No one. The insurance provided is "no fault".

○ **What do employee's gain under Workers' Compensation laws?**

No fault insurance payments for lost wages, medical care, rehabilitation, death and surviorship payments.

○ **What did the employer gain under Workers' Compensation laws?**

Limited liability and immunity from further legal actions.

O   **Under what conditions may an employer be held liable for damages despite the Workers' Compensation laws?**

Gross negligence about known hazards that resulted in damages.

O   **When were the first Workers' Compensation laws enacted?**

1911.

O   **Is the Workers' Compensation law Federally or State mandated?**

State.

O   **What career fields are exempted from Workers' Compensation?**

Farm labor, railroad employees, merchant marine, domestic service, and casual employees.

O   **What legislation is similar to Workers' Compensation for coal miners?**

Federal Coal Mine Safety and Health Act.

O   **What is the longest latency period for disease allowed for compensation by Workers' Compensation laws?**

5 years.

O   **What is the maximum time interval between exposure and filing a Workers' Compensation claim allowed by statute?**

2 years.

O   **What are "Elective Workers' Compensation Laws"?**

States that allow employers to not participate in Workman's Compensation plans at the expense of loosing the legal immunity from civil damage suits.

O   **How are most Workers' Compensation costs handled by employer's?**

Workman's compensation insurance purchasing through state or private vendors.

O   **Can a company self insure against Workers' Compensation costs?**

Yes.

O   **Who hears arguments of contested Workers' Compensation claims?**

Each state has a Workers' Compensation Board that presides over all contested cases. The decision has the effect of law, and can only be appealed by formal court hearings.

❍ **On whom is the burden of proof in contested Workers' Compensation cases?**

The employee.

❍ **Who determines the amount of loss in a Workers' Compensation case?**

Schedules of payment based on loss of function assessment, actual medical and rehabilitation costs, and a percentage of wage replacement are made by state workers' compensation boards.

❍ **What percentage wage is replaced in Workers' Compensation?**

Two-thirds.

❍ **What sponsored the largest movement in injury control device investment in the 1900's?**

Workman's Compensation "Risk Rating" that adjusts insurance premiums based on injury history of the workplace over the last 5 years.

❍ **What is the required delay prior to payment of Workers' Compensation?**

30 days.

❍ **What are the "worker incentives" for returning to work after an injury?**

Workers Compensation pays only two thirds of wage, and sponsors aggressive vocational rehabilitation.

❍ **What type of death benefits are given under Workers' Compensation?**

Funeral, burial, and payment to spouse and surviving children, until remarriage or 18 years of age respectively.

❍ **What factors are associated with Workers' Compensation case filing?**

Job dissatifaction and previous filing of a Workers' Compensation case.

❍ **What is the single greatest factor that has been shown to relate to an acute injury Workers' Compensation case becoming a chronic disability case?**

Attorney involvement. Wordall, G.D. et al.1985.

❍ **What proportion of Workers' Compensation cases are contested by the Employee?**

Fifty.

❍ **What factor has been shown to reduce the duration of Workers' Compensation claims?**

Physician attitude and focus on return to work.

❍ **What time interval away from the job is most closely correlated to permanent disability or job restriction claims?**

Six weeks.

❍ **What has the lay media termed Workers' Compensation laws?**

Compromise Laws.

❍ **What workplace practice is associated with decreased dollar and time claims under Workman's Compensation?**

Aggressive case management.

❍ **Who has the right to choose medical care location and physician under Workman's Compensation?**

The employee.

❍ **Can employers who have on-site medical staff require that all claims of injury be seen by their staff?**

No.

❍ **What rights due on-site medical services have in regards to an employee who seeks care for a Workman's Compensation case off site?**

The right to case review and management.

❍ **Do most employee's utilize the physician services suggest by the employer under Workman's Compensation cases?**

Yes.

❍ **How can Occupational Medicine services reduce Workman's Compensation claims?**

Ensure fitness for job, and aggressive case management.

❍ **Is the employer entitled to the medical information related to a Workman's Compensation case?**

Yes, in this instance it is not a breech of confidentiality to provide detailed medical information as it is pertinent to the case only.

❍ **Does Workman's Compensation cover the products used in the workplace?**

No. Product vendors are liable if any supplied material is causative to the accident and it can be proven that they were negligent.

❍ **What is the Federal System of Workers' Compensation?**

Government sponsored program that covers Federal civilians, harbor workers, longshoreman, sailors, road workers and coal miners.

❍ **Why does the federal government run a system of Workers' Compensation for non federal employee's?**

Jobs in harbors, coal mines and road repairs often contain disputes as to the state of injury, state of jurisdiction and state of intent, all of which are averted by a single federal system.

❍ **Are Airline employee's covered under the federal or state Workers' Compensation program?**

Neither.

❍ **What two things must an employee prove in order to be covered under Workers' Compensation?**

1) That they are suffering an injury or illness and 2) that it is work related.

❍ **How many disability categories are recognized by Workers' Compensation boards in all fifty states?**

Four.

❍ **Must an injury be caused by work practices in order to be covered under Workers' Compensation?**

No. The option to prove significant aggravation by work factors allows compensation of injury that was not strictly caused by work practices.

❍ **What is the most common disability classification applicable to Workers' Compensation?**

Temporary Partial.

O   **What are the defining characteristics of Temporary Partial Disability?**

Unable to perform regular duties, however able to perform some duties to maintain employment. "Light Duty"

O   **What is the 2nd most common disability category under Workman's Compensation?**

Temporary Total.

O   **What are the defining characteristics of Temporary Total Disability?**

Unable to perform any gainful employment for a short period of time, while being fully expected to return to gainful employment following a period of healing.

O   **What is the least common disability Category under Workman's Compensation?**

Permanent Total.

O   **What are the defining characteristics of Permanent Total Disability?**

Unable to return to regular gainful employment.

O   **Must a person be unable to do any income generating work in order to be classified as Permanent total disability?**

No. The law allows that some income generating work may be done, however the type or nature is unlikely to provide regular adequate income for maintenance.

O   **What is the most common long-term disability claim?**

Permanent Partial.

O   **What are the defining characteristics of Permanent Partial Disability?**

Person is expected to have a continued loss of function of some body portion that will not resolve within their lifetime.   However they are able to maintain gainful regular employment.

O   **What must an employee prove in order to substantiate a claim of Permanent Partial Disability?**

Continued loss of a body function after maximal medical improvement has been reached.

❍ **How long of a healing and treatment duration is considered adequate before pronouncing maximal medical improvement?**

One year.

❍ **Under Workman's Compensation Law, what types of medical care are allowed?**

All forms of care have been allowed, including homeopathy as long as a licensed physician "manages" and "coordinates" the care.

❍ **Are injuries arising out of travel to and from the place of work compensable?**

Yes.

❍ **Are self-inflicted injuries compensated under Workman's Compensation?**

Yes, if they are unintentional.

❍ **Are injuries that arise in the course of intoxication covered?**

No.

❍ **How long does a company have to report an employee's injury to a Workman's Compensation board?**

30 days, except in the case of death that requires reporting within 48 hours in most states.

❍ **What are the cost limits for medical care given after an injury by Workman's Compensation?**

There is no cap as to cost or duration of treatment under this regulation.

❍ **In Permanent Disability, how is the loss of income calculated?**

Based on the "Earning Capacity" which is a court determined consideration that includes willingness to work, ability to work, skill, training and the condition of the labor market at the time of injury.

❍ **Is the level of compensation equal across all of the states?**

No. The compensation level is determined on a state by state basis, with wide variations. Frequently the south eastern states pay 80 percent less benefits than the northeaster and northwestern states.

❍ **What is "Income Protection" under Workers' Compensation?**

This is a payment system that guarantees continued wage earning at the pre-injury level if a worker is unable to return to his original wage grade employment as a result of an injury. This requires return to work and a determination of Partial Permanent Disability from that type of work.

○   **What are "State Funds for a Second Injury"?**

This is a state operated fund that supports compensation for severe injuries that result in a worker with a previous assessment of permanent disability. It is a system to reduce the financial liability of employers to allow a competitive job market to exist for partially disabled workes.

○   **Is an employer required to fund vocational rehabilitation for a worker who will not ever be able to return to work within the same company or facility?**

The courts have established a "YES" in every case.

OCCUPATIONAL RELATED HEMATOLOGICAL PROBLEMS

○ **Lead impaired the synthesis of:**

Heme and to a lesser extent of globin.

○ **How does lead interfere in heme synthesis?**

By inhibiting a number of enzymes in the heme synthesis pathway.

○ **How many enzymes in the heme synthesis pathway, are inhibited by lead?**

Five enzymes

○ **What are the enzymes inhibited by lead?**

δ- aminolevulinic acid (δ-ALA) synthetase, ALA dehydrase, uroporphyrinogen decarboxylase, coproporphyrinogen oxidase, and heme synthetase (ferrochelatase).

○ **What are the by-products that might be found in the urine and serve as diagnostic aids in lead poisoning?**

ALA, coproporphyrin, and protoporphyrin.

○ **What other hematological related synthesis is impaired in lead poisoning?**

The synthesis of the enzyme pyrimidine 5' nucleotidase, which promotes the catabolism of RNA in immature red blood cells.

○ **What are the findings that can be seen in a blood smear and bone marrow respectively in lead poisoning?**

Basophilic stippling and ringed sideroblasts.

○ **What does basophilic stippling represent?**

Accumulated RNA in red blood cells.

○ **What does ringed sideroblasts represent?**

Iron- laden mitochondria located at the nuclear border of normoblasts.

O   **What type of anemia is commonly seen in lead poisoning?**

Anemia microcytic hypochromic.

O   **T/F: Hemolysis may be seen in lead poisoning.**

True.

O   **T/F: Benzene and its metabolites are bone marrow toxicant.**

False. The metabolites are toxic to the bone marrow.

O   **What are the speculated benzene metabolites responsible for its myelotoxicity?**

Phenol, hydroquinone, and benzoquinone.

O   **What are the bone marrow cell lines most susceptible to benzene?**

Erythroid, myeloid, and lymphoid.

O   **What are the hematological diseases associated with benzene?**

Aplastic anemia, myelodysplastic syndromes, and leukemia.

O   **What type of leukemia has been associated with benzene?**

Acute myeloid leukemia (AML).

O   **What is the hematological picture of aplastic anemia?**

Cytopenias.

O   **How is the bone marrow cellularity in benzene- induced aplastic anemia?**

Decreased (hypocellular bone marrow).

O   **T/F: The course of benzene- induced aplastic anemia differs from other aplastic anemias.**

False.

O   **The latency period reported between exposure and the appearance of benzene-induced AML is:**

15 - 30 years.

○ **The hematological disease(s) associated with ionizing radiation is/are:**

Leukemia, polycythemia rubra vera, and myelodysplastic syndromes.

○ **The latency period estimated between exposure to ionizing radiation and the appearance of leukemia is:**

8 to 18 years.

○ **The most frequent leukemia reported with ionizing radiation is:**

Chronic myelogenous leukemia (CML).

○ **What are the features seen in blood smears in ionizing radiation-induced leukemia:**

Neutrophils in all stages of maturation and increased numbers of basophills and eosinophills.

○ **How is the bone marrow cellularity in ionizing radiation-induced CML?**

Increased (hypercellular bone marrow).

○ **What other ancillary test/s should be done in patients with ionizing radiation- induced CML?**

Chromosomal analysis to disclose the presence of Philadelphia chromosome.

○ **What is the Philadelphia chromosome?**

The Philadelphia chromosome is a reciprocal translocation of chromosomes 9 and 22, which yields a fusion gene bcr-abl.

○ **The ultimate treatment for ionizing radiation-induced CML**

Bone marrow transplantation.

○ **The hematological effects of Arsine**

Intravascular hemolytic anemia.

○ **What are the proposed mechanisms by which arsine causes hemolytic anemia?**

Direct effect on the red blood cell.
Conversion to elemental arsenic.
Accumulation of hydrogen peroxide.

Interference with the red blood cells sodium potassium ATPase pump leading to osmotic destruction.

○ What can the blood smear may reveal in arsine-induced hemolytic anemia?

Red cell fragments, poikilocytes, red cell ghosts, and Heinz bodies.

○ What does hemoglobinuria represent in arsine-induced hemolytic anemia?

Dimmers of hemoglobin in the urine.

○ What are Heinz bodies?

Precipitated globin chains in red blood cells.

○ What markers in the plasma are elevated in arsine-induced hemolytic anemia?

Lactic dehydrogenase and unconjugated bilirubin.

○ What markers in the plasma are decreased in arsine-induced hemolytic anemia?

Haptoglobin and hemopexin.

○ What is the treatment of arsine-induced hemolytic anemia?

Removal from the exposure source, supportive care, dialysis in patients with acute oliguric renal failure, and exchange transfusion to remove irreversibly damaged and arsenic-bearing red blood cells.

○ What other chemicals may cause hemolytic anemia?

Naphthalene (moth balls), methylene chloride, zineb (zinc ethylene-bis-dithiocarbamate), chlorates (ClO3).

○ What is the hematological effect of trimellitic anhydride (TMA)?

Immune- related hemolytic anemia.

○ What is methemoglobin?

Hemoglobin in which the iron molecule has been oxidized to Fe^{+3} (ferric state)

○ What does the presence of methemoglobin do to the hemoglobin dissociation curve?

Shifts the curve to the left.

❍ **What is the significance of a "left shifted" curve?**

High affinity of hemoglobin to oxygen leading to decreased release to the tissues.

❍ **Is methemoglobin capable of carry oxygen?**

No.

❍ **Does the human body normally create methemoglobin?**

Yes, this occurs as a result of an electron loss from iron to oxygen.

❍ **What is the baseline level of methemoglobin in a healthy person?**

Less than 1%.

❍ **How does the iron normally convert back to the ferrous state?**

By the enzyme NADH dependent methemoglobin reductase.

❍ **From what metabolic pathway the NADH is derived in NADH dependent methemoglobin reductase?**

From glycolisis.

❍ **What is the common denominator between hemolysis and methemoglobinemia?**

The causative agents, which induce both an oxidative stress to the red blood cells and methemoglobinemia.

❍ **Who are particularly more prone to develop hemolysis?**

Patients with G6PD deficiency.

❍ **What are the first symptoms of significant methemoglobinemia?**

Dyspnea, fatigue, headache, and dizziness.

❍ **At what level of methemoglobin is cyanosis usually seen?**

15-20%.

❍ **What characteristics may one observe when drawing a blood sample from a patient with significant methemoglobinemia?**

"Chocolate brown" color of the blood.

○   **What value of oxygen saturation the pulse oxymeter will show in a patient with methemoglobinemia?**

85%.

○   **What chemical agents (not medications) may cause methemoglobinemia and in higher doses also hemolysis?**

Aniline dyes, cresol, naphthalene, nitrobenzene, phenol, and phenylsemicarbazide.

○   **Why may infants less than four months of age be more susceptible to methemoglobinemia?**

The enzyme NADH methemoglobin reductase does not reach full activity level around this age.

○   **What is the antidote for methemoglobinemia?**

Methylene blue.

○   **T/F: Methylene blue is considered a reducing agent.**

False. Methylene blue is an <u>oxidative agent</u> but its metabolite, leukomethylene blue, is considered a reducing agent.

○   **How does methylene blue help to reduce methemoglobin?**

Methylene blue is converted to leukomethylene blue by NADPH methemoglobin reductase. The leulomethylene blue then reduces the methemoglobin.

○   **From what metabolic pathway the NADPH is derived in NADPH methemoglobin reductase?**

From the hexose monophosphate pathway.

○   **Why might methylene blue be ineffective in patients with G6PD deficiency?**

Because they are unable to generate NADPH in the red blood cell which is necessary for NADPH methemoglobin reductase to convert methylene blue to leukomethylene blue.

○   **What are the indications for methylene blue therapy?**

It is indicated in any patient with symptomatic methemoglobinemia.

○   **What are the potentially side effects of methylene blue?**

Paradoxical methemoglobinemia and hemolysis.

○ **What are the porphyrias?**

Porphyrias are a group of diseases that result from defective heme biosynthesis with subsequently accumulation of heme precursors. These are divided in primary (hereditary) and acquired (due to chemical exposures).

○ **Clinically, the acquired porphyrias are similar to what hereditary type?**

Porphyria cutanea tarda.

○ **To what group the acquired porphyrias belong?**

Hepatic porphyrias.

○ **What are the clinical manifestations of the acquired porphyrias?**

Cutaneous photosensitivity manifested as the presence of fluid filled vesicles and bullae in sun-exposed areas with occasionally hypertrichosis and hyperpigmentation especially of the face; hepatomegaly; and impaired heme synthesis.

○ **What substances have been associated with the acquired porphyrias?**

Aluminum; 2- Benzyl-4,6- dichlorophenol; 0- Benzyl- p- chlorophenol; hexachlorobenzene; 2,3, 7,8- Tetrachlorodibenzo-p- dioxin; 2,4- Dichlorophenol; 2,4,5- Trichlorophenol.

○ **The activity of what enzyme is decreased in the acquired porphyrias?**

Uroporphyrinogen (URO) decarboxylase.

○ **Chemical agents associated with agranulocytosis and neutropenia.**

Antimony, arsenic, benzene, DDT, dinitrophenol, gold salts, thioglycolic acid (cold wave).

○ **What agents have been associated with immune- mediated thrombocytopenia?**

Toluene diisocyanate and turpentine.

○ **Anticoagulants might be found in the industry of:**

Rodenticides.

○ **With what common name are the anticoagulant rodenticides well known?**

They are commonly known as superwarfarin rodenticides.

❍ **What is the mechanism of action of the superwarfarins?**

They inhibit vitamin K 2,3 epoxide reductase and to a lesser extent, also vitamin K quinone reductase.

❍ **What coagulation factors are inhibited by the super- warfarins?**

Vitamin K dependent coagulation factor 10, 9,7, and 2.

❍ **What is sulfhemoglobin?**

Sulfhemoglobin is a green-pigmented molecule containing a sulfur atom instead of an iron atom inside the porphyrin ring.

❍ **Exposure to what chemical may induce sulfhemoglobinemia?**

Exposure to hydrogen sulfide gas.

❍ **What does carbon monoxide do to the hemoglobin dissociation curve?**

It shifts it to the left.

OCCUPATIONAL RELATED HEPATIC PROBLEMS

○ **In how many categories toxic liver disorders can be divided?**

Three categories according to their etiology: viral hepatitis, chemical- induced hepatitis, and physical agent- induced lesions.

○ **What is the predominant cause of morbidity in the hepatology clinical practice?**

Inflammatory liver disease.

○ **What is the primary etiology of hepatic inflammation?**

Infectious primarily by viruses.

○ **What are the common known viruses, which cause hepatitis?**

Hepatitis A virus, hepatitis B virus, hepatitis C virus, hepatitis D virus, hepatitis E virus, Epstein-Barr virus, and cytomegalovirus. (CMV)

○ **Which hepatitis virus has not been identified so far in the USA as a cause of hepatitis?**

Hepatitis E.

○ **What is the most common hepatitis encountered in health care workers?**

Hepatitis B and C.

○ **What are the three general patterns, which follow chemical –induced hepatic injury?**

Cytotoxic injury, cholestatic injury, and mixed cytotoxic and cholestatic injury.

○ **What are the different identified mechanisms of liver toxicity?**

Lipid peroxidation, reactive oxygen species formation, covalent binding to liver proteins, gluthatione depletion, peroxisome proliferation, interference with protein synthesis, plasma membrane damage, and cytokine induced.

○ **What are the routes by which toxicants may reach the liver?**

Inhalation, dermal, and oral.

○ **How is the portal triad composed?**

The triad is composed by the hepatic artery, portal vein, and the bile duct.

○ **What is the liver acinus?**

The acinus is the functional unit of the liver.

○ **Into how many zones is the acinus divided?**

In three zones: zone I or periportal area, zone II or the intermediate area, and zone III or centrilobular area around the hepatic vein.

○ **What zone is toxicologically highly important?**

Zone III.

○ **Why does zone III constitute the most important area in toxicology?**

Because it contains the enzymes of the cytochrome P-450 system responsible for the metabolism of drugs and chemical substances.

○ **What are phase I and II reactions?**

These are reactions taking place in the liver, which make compounds more excretable and sometimes less toxic.

○ **Where do phase I reactions take place?**

They take place at zone III.

○ **How anatomically can hepatic injury manifest?**

Hepatic injury from any source can manifest as steatosis, necrosis, cholestasis, fibrosis, and cirrhosis.

○ **How is steatosis defined morphologically?**

Steatosis is defined morphologically as greater than 5% hepatocytes containing fat, or as greater than 5g lipid per 100 g hepatic tissue.

○ **How steatosis is divided?**

Steatosis is divided to macro and microsteatosis.

○ **What drugs/ substances may cause macrosteatosis?**

Ethanol and corticosteroids.

○ **What drugs have been associated with microsteatosis?**

Valproic acid and tetracycline.

○ **Drugs/ substances, which cause zone III necrosis**

Acetaminophen and carbon tetrachloride. (CCl_4)

○ **Drugs/ substances, which cause preferentially zone I necrosis**

Iron and isoniazide.

○ **What antibiotics may cause cholestatic injury?**

Erythomycin and augmentin.

○ **What chemical has been associated with angiosarcoma of the liver?**

Vinyl chloride.

○ **Fungi derived substance associated with hepatocellular carcinoma.**

Aflatoxin.

○ **What chemicals have been reportedly associated with hepatic steatosis?**

Chlorinated and aromatic hydrocarbons (e.g. carbon tetrachloride), hydrazine derivatives, and phosphorus.

○ **What chemicals have been associated with liver cholestasis?**

Methylenediamine, toluene diisocyanate, and paraquat.

○ **Metal(s) associated with liver cirrhosis**

Arsenic.

○ **Substances associated with hepatocellular carcinoma**

Aflatoxins, plant alkaloids, pyrrolizidine alkaloids (cycasin, safrole), nitrosamines, nitrosamides, heterocyclic aromatic amines, ethanol, androgen- anabolic steroids, and azo dyes.

○ **Into what major categories may hepatotoxins be divided?**

In two categories: predictable (intrinsic) and unpredictable (idiosyncratic).

○ **T/F: Idiosyncratic hepatic injury is dose-dependent.**

False.

○ **T/F: Liver injury associated to intrinsic hepatotoxins is dose dependent.**

True.

○ **How many possible mechanisms of idiosyncratic liver injury are known?**

Two, hypersensitivity and metabolic aberration.

○ **What are the characteristics of a hypersensitivity injury?**

Systemic symptoms such as fever and rash, peripheral eosinophilia, and liver histology supporting hypersensitivity (Eosinophils, granulomatous inflammatory infiltration).

○ **What anticonvulsant drug may cause a hypersensitivity idiosyncratic liver injury?**

Phenytoin. *(Dilantin)*

○ **Aliphatic hydrocarbons associated with occupational liver injury**

Alicyclic hydrocarbons, e.g. cyclopropane; n-heptane, and turpentine.

○ **Alcohols associated with occupational liver injury**

Allyl alcohol, ethyl alcohol, ethylene chlorohydrin, methyl alcohol, and ethylene glycol ethers.

○ **Ethers and epoxy compounds associated with occupational liver injury**

Dioxane, epichlorohydrin, ethylene oxide, ethyl ether.

○ **Pesticide associated with liver injury and male infertility**

Dibromochloropropane (DBCP).

○ **Pesticides associated with liver injury**

Bipyridyls, thallium sulfate, kepone (chlordecone), and arsenic.

❍ **Chemical substance used in dry-cleaning processes associated with liver injury**

Perchloroethylene.

❍ **What type of liver injury is associated with chloroform?**

Steatosis and zone III necrosis.

❍ **Liver injury associated with repeated exposures to trichloroethylene**

Centrilobular (zone III) necrosis.

❍ **T/F: Drug induced hepatocellular injury resembles clinically and in laboratory to viral hepatitis clinically.**

True.

❍ **What liver enzymes are expected to be elevated in hepatocellular injury?**

ALT, AST, and to some degree alkaline phosphatase.

❍ **What liver enzymes are elevated in cholestatic injury?**

Alkaline phosphatase and γ glutaryl transferase.

❍ **What liver enzyme is considered to be more "liver specific": ALT or AST?**

ALT.

❍ **How are the liver enzymes in steatotic liver?**

The ALT, AST, and alkaline phosphatase could be normal or mildly elevated.

❍ **What bilirubin fraction is usually elevated in hepatocellular injury?**

The direct bilirubin > indirect bilirubin.

❍ **What the direct bilirubin represents?**

It represents conjugated bilirubin.

❍ **What condition may lead to indirect hyperbilirubinemia?**

Hemolysis.

○ **What enzyme(s) can be elevated in hemolysis and drug-induced liver injury?**

Total lactate dehydrogenase.

○ **What is the most specific enzyme to detect biliary tract disease?**

5'- Nucleotidase.

○ **Identify the etiology of the hepatitis: IgM anti-HAV positive, IgG anti HAV negative**

Recent hepatitis A.

○ **HBsAg negative, HBsAb positive, anti-HBc positive**

Acute viral hepatitis B.

○ **HBsAg positive, HBsAb positive, anti-HBc positive, HBV DNA undetectable, HBeAg negative**

This situation does not exist because HBV DNA is positive in chronic hepatitis B.

○ **HBsAg positive, HBsAb positive, anti-HBc positive, HBV DNA positive, HBeAg negative**

Chronic Hepatitis B, non-replicating phase.

○ **HBsAg positive, HBsAb positive, anti-HBc positive, HBV DNA positive, HBeAg positive**

Chronic Hepatitis B, replicating phase.

○ **Anti HCV positive**

Hepatitis C.

○ **What metallic compounds have been identified as hepatotoxins?**

Arsenic, beryllium, bismuth, boron, cadmium, chromium, copper, germanium, carbonyls (metal), iron, nickel, thallium, selenium, thorium dioxide, tin, and uranium.

○ **What epoxy resin hardener has been associated with cholestatic injury?**

Methylene dianiline.

○ **The term Spanish toxic oil syndrome refers to:**

Chronic cholestatic liver disease induced by ingestion of adulterated denatured rapeseed oil.

○ **What is the liver injury encountered with exposure to yellow phosphorus?**

Steatosis and necrosis.

○ **What type of liver injury has been associated with occupational exposures to styrene, toluene, and trichloroethane?**

Liver steatosis.

○ **What type of liver injury was found in the munitions industry and what was the allegedly causative agent?**

Liver steatosis and necrosis, trinitrotoluene (TNT).

○ **Chemical substance associated with liver injury found in fabric coating factory.**

Dimethylformamide (DMF).

○ **What chemical(s) has (ve) been associated with hepatoportal sclerosis?**

Vinyl chloride in polyvinyl chloride polymerization manufacturing plants, inorganic arsenic, and thorium compounds.

○ **What chemicals have been reportedly associated with fulminant hepatic failure?**

TNT, CCl4, chloroform, trichloroethylene, and 2- nitropropane.

○ **What industries/workplaces have been associated with a high prevalence of liver cirrhosis among workers?**

Shipyard, printers, munitions, pesticide industry, fuel refineries, anesthesiologists, morticians, electrical capacitors industry.

○ **What substances have been associated with porphyria cutanea tarda?**

Vinyl chloride, methyl chloride, hexachlorobenzene, and tetrachlordibenzo-p-dioxin (TCDD).

○ **What type of hepatic injury may be encounter in heat stroke?**

Centrilobular necrosis and cholestasis.

○ **What is the dose of ionizing radiation necessary to induce radiation hepatitis?**

3,000 to 6,000 rads.

○   **What is the elapsed time from radiation exposure to hepatic injury?**

Two to six weeks.

○   **What is the hepatic injury seen in radiation hepatitis?**

Fibrosis, cirrhosis, obliteration of the central vein, and centrilobular congestion.

OCCUPATIONAL RELATED RENAL PROBLEMS

❍ **T/F: Occupational and environmental causes are included in the United States Renal Data System Report.**

False.

❍ **What is the sensitivity of the urine dipstick in identifying hematuria?**

Greater than 90%.

❍ **How is hematuria defined?**

Hematuria is defined as the presence of 3 or more erythrocytes/HPF of centrifuged sediment examined microscopically.

❍ **How can hematuria be differentiated from hemoglobinuria?**

By microscopic examination of the urine with identification of erythrocytes in the urine.

❍ **How chemically-associated urinary tract neoplasms may present?**

They may present as hematuria.

❍ **What are the etiologies for nephrogenic (as compared with urologic) hematuria?**

Glomerular (glomerulopathies) and non- glomerular (tubulointerstitial, renovascular, and systemic).

❍ **What characterizes the glomerular hematurias?**

The presence of red blood cell casts.

❍ **T/F: Single use of a non steroidal anti-inflammatory drugs (NSAID) may cause papillary necrosis in the kidney.**

False. Chronic use.

❍ **What is the etiology of papillary necrosis?**

Ischemia to the collecting ducts.

○   **What are the pyelographic findings of papillary necrosis?**

Contrast dye pooling in the defect resulting from the sloughed papilla.

○   **What renal disease has been associated with exposure to hydrocarbon solvents?**

Glomerulonephritis.

○   **How is proteinuria defined?**

Proteinuria is defined as the excretion of 150 mg or more of albumin in the urine in a 24 hours period.

○   **What is the daily normal urinary protein excretion?**

150 mg.

○   **How is nephrotic- ranged proteinuria defined?**

Nephrotic ranged proteinuria is defined as the excretion of ≥ 3 grams of protein in the urine in a 24 hours period or of >3.5 g per 1.73 m2 per 24 hours.

○   **Above what protein daily amount in the urine the urine dipstick becomes positive?**

Above 300 mg.

○   **How is nephrotic syndrome defined?**

Nephrotic syndrome is defined as nephritic range proteinuria accompanied with hypoalbuminemia, edema, hyperlipidemia, lipiduria, and hypercoagulability.

○   **How lipiduria is seen when the urine is examined under a polarization microscopy?**

As small droplets which deflects light in the pattern of Maltese cross.

○   **What are oval fat bodies?**

Are macrophages with phagocitized fat droplets.

○   **What is the estimated number of workers potentially exposed to nephrotoxic chemicals?**

Four millions.

❍ **T/F: The mortality from renal diseases in cohorts of workers exposed to lead and cadmium is higher than the general population.**

True.

❍ **How can chemicals affect the renal function or structures?**

By having a direct effect on the different kidney structures or indirectly by causing intravascular hemolysis, rhabdomyolisis, or cardiac failure.

❍ **What metals have been associated with acute or chronic renal damage in humans?**

Arsenic, bismuth, chromium, cadmium, copper, germanium, gold, lithium, mercury, platinum, silver, thalium, uranium.

❍ **What type of mercury has been classically described as nephrotoxic?**

Inorganic mercury.

❍ **What type of injury does inorganic mercury typically cause to the kidneys?**

Acute tubular necrosis. *(ATN)*

❍ **T/F: *(Organic)* Methyl mercury is nephrotoxic as inorganic mercury.**

False.

❍ **T/F: Ethyl and phenyl mercury are nephrotoxic as inorganic mercury.**

True.

❍ **What chlorinated hydrocarbons have been associated with acute or chronic renal damage?**

Carbon tetrachloride, 1,2- Dichloromethane (methylene chloride), trichloroethylene, chloroform, hexachloro-1,3-butadiene, dichloracetylene, perchloroethylene, trichloroethane.

❍ **What aromatic, non-halogenated hydrocarbons have been associated with acute and chronic renal damage?**

Toluene and Styrene.

❍ **What part of the nephron might be damaged in chronic exposure to toluene?**

Tubulointerstitial cells.

❍ **What renal disease has been associated with chronic toluene exposure?**

Type I (distal) renal tubular acidosis.

❍ **What laboratory tests are necessary to diagnose renal tubular acidosis?**

Urine pH and serum electrolytes.

❍ **What do the laboratory tests show in distal RTA?**

Hypokalemia, hyperchloremia, normal anion gap metabolic acidosis, and urine pH> 6.0.

❍ **How can workers be monitored for chronic toluene exposure?**

By measuring urine concentrations of hippuric acid.

❍ **What other industrial chemicals have been associated with renal injury?**

Ethylene glycol, diethylene glycol, ethylene glycol ethers (in high doses), carbon disulfide, dioxane.

❍ **What low molecular weight proteins may appear in early stages of lead nephropathy?**

Beta-2 microglobulin, retinol- binding protein (RBP), and N-acetyl- β-D- glucosaminidase (NAG).

❍ **How can low molecular weight proteins be distinguished from albumin or other high molecular weight proteins?**

By urinary protein electrophoresis.

❍ **What type of glomerulopathy has been associated with inhalation of hydrocarbon solvents?**

Rapidly progressive glomerulonephritis (RPGN).

❍ **What is the histology pattern described in RPGN?**

Subepithelial crescentic glomerular injury.

❍ **What is the type of immune injury described in hydrocarbons-related RPGN?**

Immune complex related and production of antiglomerular basement antibody which binds to the glomerular basement membrane.

❍ **T/F: Exposure to high dose mercury vapors may damage the tubular cells.**

True.

○ **Can early tubular injury be measured?**

Yes.

○ **Can early tubular injury be detected?**

Yes.

○ **What is the most common index measured in the urine to detect early tubular injury?**

N-acetyl- β-D- glucosaminidase (NAG).

○ **What part of the nephron is classically injured in lead nephropathy?**

The proximal tubule.

○ **How is the renal syndrome caused by chronic lead exposure termed?**

Fanconi-like syndrome.

○ **What are the renal clinical manifestations of the Fanconi-like syndrome?**

Aminoaciduria, glycosuria, bicarbonaturia, phosphaturia, uric-aciduria.

○ **What microscopic findings are seen in the kidneys, in the Fanconi-like syndrome?**

Cytosolic and nuclear inclusion bodies.

○ **What do inclusion bodies represent?**

They represent a lead-protein complex which were taken up by endocytosis by the tubular cells.

○ **T/F: Lead may also cause glomerular damage.**

False.

○ **T/F: There is a direct correlation between blood lead levels and the severity of lead nephropathy.**

False.

○ **What type of renal tubular acidosis (RTA) may patients with Fanconi-like syndrome develop?**

RTA type II (proximal type).

○ **How does lead impair Vitamin D synthesis?**

By preventing the hydroxylation of 25- hydroxyvitamin D to 1,25 dehydroxy- vitamin D.

○ **How does lead prevent the hydroxylation of 25- hydroxyvitamin D?**

Lead inhibits the heme-contained enzyme responsible for the hydroxylation.

○ **T/F: Cadmium may lead to end stage renal disease.**

True.

○ **What are the nephron parts affected by cadmium?**

Renal tubular cells and glomeruli.

○ **What is the critical concentration of cadmium in the renal cortex that produces tubular dysfunction?**

In 10 % of the population is 200 μg/g and in 50 % of the population is 300μg/g.

○ **How is renal tubular damage initially reflected in cadmium-induced nephropathy?**

Tubular damage is initially reflected by low molecular weight proteinuria.

○ **What does the finding of low molecular weight proteinuria represent?**

It represents renal tubular damage.

○ **What does the finding of high molecular weight (albumin, trasferin) proteinuria represent?**

It represents glomerular leak or in other words, glomerular damage.

○ **What is the pathogenesis of the glomerular lesions induced by cadmium?**

The pathogenesis is presently unknown.

○ **T/F: There is a correlation between urinary cadmium concentrations and the severity or renal injury.**

True.

O   **How does cadmium circulate in the blood?**

Cadmium circulates in the blood bound to metallothionein protein.

O   **The metabolism of what cation is affected by cadmium?**

Calcium.

O   **What is the half life of cadmium in the kidneys?**

The half life of cadmium in the kidneys may exceed 15 years.

O   **What chelation therapy is considered efficient for chronic cadmium poisoning?**

None.

O   **What other organ might be affected in chronic cadmium poisoning?**

The skeleton.

O   **What are the skeletal changes in chronic cadmium poisoning?**

Bone pain, osteoporosis and osteomalacia.

O   **What type of chromium has been associated with renal injury?**

Hexavalent chromium (chromate and dichromate).

O   **What type of renal injury has been associated with silica?**

Glomerulonephritis.

O   **What biological agents have been associated with renal failure?**

Mycotoxins.

O   **What mycotoxins have been associated with renal injury and failure?**

Ochratoxin A, fumonisins, and aristolochic acid.

O   **What is the renal disease associated with exposure to formaldehyde?**

Membranous glomerulonephritis.

❍ **What renal disease has been associated in dye workers?**

Bladder cancer.

❍ **What is the renal disease associated with lithium?**

Nephrogenic diabetes insipidus.

❍ **What herbicide is associated with acute renal failure?**

Paraquat (paraquat is a tubular toxin).

❍ **What is the renal disease associated with gold?**

Membranous glomerulonephritis.

❍ **What are the clinical manifestations of membranous glomerulonephritis?**

Nephrotic- ranged proteinuria and nephrotic syndrome.

REGULATORY ISSUES

○   **The United States legal system is primarily a conflation of principles from what two historical legal systems?**

Roman civil law, which was based on a statutory code.
English common law, which was based on precedent (previous court decisions in similar cases).

○   **In which state does the legal system rely heavily upon a separate historical tradition?**

Louisiana, where much of the legal system has evolved from the French Napoleonic Code.

○   **The authority to pass laws and regulations is generally considered to come from two basic powers, police power and parens patriae. What is the difference between these two justifications for establishing and applying legal power?**

Police power refers to the right of the state to protect public health, welfare, safety, and morals. In other words, it is the right of the state to protect society as a whole. Parens patriae, meaning the state acting as parent, applies to the right of the state to protect people who are unable to take care of themselves. That is, it is the right of the state to protect individuals rather than society at large

○   **Parens patriae is not restricted to the mentally ill or mentally disabled. Give an example of legislation based upon police power vs. legislation based upon parens patriae for ordinary citizens.**

Many examples could be given, and legislation may be based upon both principles. Prohibition of school attendance for those with certain communicable diseases would be an example of police power, since the individual whose activities are being regulated is already sick and it is the public that is being protected. Laws against riding a motorcycle without a helmet are designed primarily to protect individuals from their own actions and thus would be considered to be based upon parens patriae. Gun-control legislation and laws against driving while intoxicated are designed to protect both society and the individual and have elements of both police power and parens patriae.

○   **What are the prime constitutional tests of the legitimacy of a law based upon police power?**

There must be a legitimate interest (that is, a reasonable relationship between the proscribed behavior and public safety or interest must exist), and in the case of interference with a fundamental right of an individual, the state must demonstrate a compelling interest.

❍   **The U.S. Constitution includes both a commerce clause and also a taxing and spending power. How do these clauses affect the right of the federal government to pass laws?**

The commerce clause allows the federal government to enact laws affecting interstate commerce and is the basis for federal regulation of environmental health, health care, and sanitation, among other things. The taxing and spending authority allows the Congress to grant or withhold funds to states.

❍   **Where in the U.S. Constitution do the commerce-regulatory authority and taxing authority appear?**

Section 8 of Article 2.

❍   **What two types of suits can be brought in U.S. courts, and what is the difference between them?**

Civil suits, brought by private citizens (plaintiffs) against one or more defendants to determine liability and resulting, through a court judgment, in the issuance of a court order or declaration or in the awarding of damages.

Criminal suits, brought by a local or state government or the federal government by means of a prosecutor against a defendant to determine guilt for the purpose of punishment or deterrence and resulting in a fine or imprisonment.

❍   **What is the difference in burden of proof between a civil suit and a criminal suit?**

In a civil suit, proof is considered to be a preponderance of evidence, that is, a condition in which it is "more probable than not" that the event in question occurred. In a criminal suit, the event must be proved "beyond a reasonable doubt."

❍   **Two important branches of law are tort law and contract law. What is a tort?**

A legally redressable civil wrong consisting of an injury to person, property, or reputation. The perpetrator of the injury is called the tortfeasor.

❍   **What kinds of liability exist in tort cases?**

Strict liability (in which no fault is required).
Negligence (failure to exercise reasonable caution), including malpractice (failure to act as a reasonable prudent professional would act).
Gross negligence (willful or reckless disregard of others).
Intentional liability (deliberate injury).

❍ **Intentional, or deliberate, torts may include battery (intentional bodily contact without permission), fraud or deceit, and breach of confidentiality. What kinds of breaches of confidentiality exist in tort law?**

Breach of an implied contract.
Invasion of privacy.
Unprofessional conduct.
Defamation of character.
Bad faith breach of conduct (which may convert a tort to a contract action).

❍ **Under what category of tort could a suit be brought against a physician who fails to provide informed consent to a patient?**

Battery.

❍ **Occupational healthcare providers may become tortfeasors by reason of negligence. What are the four Ds required to demonstrate negligence in a tort case?**

Duty: the presence of an obligation or standard of care.
Dereliction of duty: Performance significantly below the standard of care.
Damage: Physical injury, psychological harm, or loss of reputation. (Economic loss is not recoverable if it is the sole loss.)
Direct causation: Negligence must represent the proximate cause of the damage.

❍ **Institutions may become liable through a principle called vicarious liability for torts committed by their healthcare-provider employees. What two types of vicarious liability exist?**

Respondeat superior ("let the master answer"): An employer is normally liable for actions of employers acting as agents for the employer in the normal scope of employment.
Apparent (ostensible) liability: An organization may be liable for the actions of independent contractors if they appear to be employees.

❍ **So-called "toxic torts," brought against organizations to recover damages from environmental release of toxicants, can be based upon strict liability (in highly hazardous industries), negligence, breach of expressed or implied warranty, or intentional misconduct. What kinds of damages have been recovered in toxic-tort cases?**

Usual damages (e.g., medical expenses, lost earnings, and pain and suffering).
Future risk of illness (documentation of exposure alone may suffice in some cases).
Fear of future illness (the fact of exposure plus a "serious, reasonable, and genuine fear").
Cost of medical surveillance (e.g., "response costs" from CERCLA).

❍ **In contract law, what is a contract?**

A consensual agreement (either expressed or implied) between two or more parties whereby each undertakes defined obligations to the other.

❍   **In general, what kinds of damages can be awarded in a contract case?**

Tangible economic losses (not emotional distress or other intangible harms, and in most cases not punitive damages).

❍   **A specific kind of breach of contract is breach of warranty, in which economic losses from a bad outcome can be awarded despite lack of negligence. How significant of a problem is this for medical-malpractice cases involving occupational healthcare providers?**

The courts have generally been reluctant to apply breach of warranty to cases of medical malpractice.

❍   **In general medical practice, when a physician begins seeing a patient an implied contract is presumed to have occurred. What factors help determine whether an occupational healthcare provider has established a contract with an ill or injured worker?**

Whether the provider is treating or just examining the worker.
For whose benefit the provider is providing the service.
The period during which the provider sees the worker.
Reasonable expectations of the provider and the worker.
The nature of the worker's consent to the examination.

❍   **What are the duties of a physician if a contractual relationship (that is, a physician-patient, or physician-worker, relationship) with a worker exists?**

Informing the worker of his or her medical condition and pertinent facts about that condition.
Notifying the worker of any test results and diagnoses.
Informing the worker of the need for treatment.
Giving the worker instructions for self-care.
Advising the worker of any aggravating conditions.
Preserving the confidentiality of the worker's condition.
Referring the worker to a specialist if appropriate.

❍   **What acrostic can be used as a mnemonic device to help remember these essential duties of a physician with an express or implied contract with a worker?**

MANIACS:
M: Medical condition.
A: Any test results.
N: Need for treatment.
I: Instructions for self-care.
A: Aggravating conditions.
C: Confidentiality.
S: Specialist referral.

❍ **If an occupational healthcare provider has not established a contractual physician-patient with a worker, what then are the provider responsibilities under the law?**

Some courts hold that the only legal responsibility is primum non nocere ("first, do no harm"). Thus, an independent medical examiner without a contractual relationship with a worker is exempt from legal immunity if he or she causes injury to the patient during the course of the examination. Other courts have held that the provider has a legal responsibility to exercise some reasonable care. If personal medical advice is given during the course of a visit, a contractual relationship, with all of its attendant provider responsibilities, is usually held to have been established.

❍ **If an occupational healthcare provider is an independent contractor and makes a negligent medical assessment resulting in an improper job placement, is the provider immune from prosecution under contract law?**

No.

❍ **What information from a medical examination can legally be communicated to an employer?**

Information relating to the employee's ability to perform the essential functions of the job. Other medical diagnoses and findings are not to be reported.

❍ **Can an occupational-healthcare professional be legally compelled to perform medical testing relating to the arrest and prosecution of a worker?**

No.

 ❍ **Is infection of a worker with human immunodeficiency virus (HIV) a disease that has been mandated at the federal level as reportable to the National Notifiable Diseases Surveillance System (NNDSS)?**

No; pediatric HIV infection is a reportable infectious disease, but HIV infection in adults is not. In addition, reporting to the NNDSS by states is voluntary.

❍ **T/F: When an overriding compelling interest dictates that a physician report a disease or other condition in a patient (including a worker), the physician must by law inform the patient that the condition is being reported.**

False.

❍ **Is a regulation a law?**

Yes; all regulations are laws (or have the force of law, which amounts to the same thing), but not all laws are regulations.

○   **What is the difference between a statute and a regulation?**

A statute is a law enacted by a representative legislature (as opposed to a fiat decree issuing from a monarch) and may be stated in broad general terms. (Statues enacted by city or county legislative bodies are usually called ordinances.) A regulation, sometimes also called a rule and in some contexts a standard, is a governmental order (in some contexts called an executive order) with the force of law. It usually deals with specific details of a broad law. For example, the Occupational Safety and Health Act (OSH Act) is a statutory law designed to protect workers but does not in itself specify the maximal permissible blood levels of lead in a worker. This detail appears in one of many regulations issued to support the general law.

○   **The three well-known divisions of the U.S. federal governmental are the legislative, executive, and judicial branches. What responsibility does each branch have regarding laws?**

The legislative branch enacts laws (statutes), the executive branch enforces laws, and the judicial branch interprets laws.

○   **Many administrative agencies exist within the U.S. federal government. What are their responsibilities concerning federal regulations?**

They are entitled to enact, enforce, and interpret federal rules and regulations (they may also grant licenses).

○   **With which branch or branches of the federal government are U.S. administrative agencies grouped?**

Some fall under the executive branch; others are independent agencies.

○   **What is the difference between the content of the U.S. Code (USC) and the Code of Federal Regulations (CFR)?**

The USC, published every six years, contains laws passed by the Congress; the CFR contains regulations (Rules) made by federal agencies and executive departments (see http://www.findlaw.com/casecode). The CFR is an annual publication with none of the so-called "pocket parts" of the USC, there is no annotated version of the CFR (with case notes and legal-review citations) as is the case with the USC, and the regulations in the CFR tend to be more detailed than the statutory laws of the USC.

○   **What is the difference between the Code of Federal Regulations (CFR) and the Federal Register?**

The CFR is a list of finalized federal rules, or regulations. The Federal Register is a daily publication containing new rules, proposed rules, and notices from federal agencies and executive departments as well as executive orders and other presidential documents. Finalized items from the Federal Register are eventually incorporated into new editions of the CFR.

○   **A law from the USC may have the format 15 USC 1414 (1988), referring to a law found in Section 1414 of Title 15 of the 1988 edition of the USC. A regulation from the CFR may be cited as, for example, 47 CFR 64.1200 (2001), meaning Section 64.1200 of Volume 47 of the 2001 edition of the CFR. There is yet another way of referring to certain laws. What does the PL in PL 91-173 (the Mine Safety and Health Act) represent?**

Public Law. Public laws are laws signed by the president. The number appearing between PL and the hyphen in the citation of the law refers to the Congress that passed the law, and the next number has reference to the chronology of the laws passed during that Congress; thus PL 91-173 was the 173rd statute enacted by the 91st Congress. Public laws are known as "slip laws" until they are compiled into the Statutes at Large at the end of a session of the Congress. They then are referred to as "session laws" until they become part of the USC. Citations of session laws include "Stat," as in the fictitious example 99 Stat 2234 (1973), in which 99, 2234, and (1973) refer to the volume number, page number, and year of passage of the law, respectively.

○   **The Occupational Safety and Health Act of 1970 (OSH Act), originally PL 91-596 and now 29 USC 651 et seq., was enacted "to assure so far as possible every working man and woman in the Nation safe and healthful working conditions" [29 USC 651(b)]. In addition to providing a safe and healthful workplace, what other principal functions does the OSH Act assign to the Occupational Safety and Health Administration (OSHA)?**

Setting standards and conducting workplace inspections.

○   **Coverage under the OSH Act is extended to employers and employees in all 50 U.S. states, the District of Columbia, Puerto Rico, and all other federal territories by mean of what agency or agencies?**

The Secretary of the Department of Labor has delegated authority under the OSH Act to the Assistant Secretary for Occupational Safety and Health, who heads the Occupational Safety and Health Administration (OSHA). However, states may institute their own job safety and health programs as long as those programs are approved by OSHA and include regulations at least as stringent as those promulgated by OSHA itself.

○   **Does the OSH Act consider religious groups to be employers?**

Yes, to the extent that they employ workers for secular purposes.

○   **What are exclusions to coverage under the OSH Act?**

Self-employed workers.
Farms at which only immediate family members of the farmer are employed.

Employment settings (such as mining, nuclear energy, and some cases of transportation industries) already covered by other federal regulatory agencies.
Employees of state and local governments in states with their own OSHA-approved safety and health programs.

○ **What are the four main types of industries subject to OSHA regulations?**

General industry (covered by 29 CFR 1910).
Construction (covered by 29 CFR 1926).
Maritime industries, including shipyards, marine terminals, and longshoring (covered by 29 CFR 1915 through 1919).
Agriculture (covered by 29 CFR 1928).

○ **Is 29 CFR 1910 the same as 29 USC 1910?**

No. 29 USC 1910 does not in fact exist.

○ **Federally mandated occupational-safety-and-health standards for general industry can be found in 29 CFR 1910, which has twenty-six subparts, labeled A through Z. Subparts U, V, X, and Y are blank. Why?**

They are set aside for future regulations.

○ **Subpart H (containing Sections 101 through 120) of the 29 CFR 1910 contains regulations for hazardous materials. What topic is regulated by the very last subpart, Subpart Z (containing Sections 1000 through 1500) of 29 CFR 1910?**

"Toxic and Hazardous Substances," meaning mostly air contaminants, mineral dusts (including asbestos), bloodborne pathogens, and certain specific chemicals as opposed to the treatment in Subpart H of compressed gases, explosive hazards, and process requirements for highly hazardous chemicals in general.

○ **Where in 29 CFR 1910 is the so-called "general duty clause" of OSHA?**

Nowhere. It can be found in Section 5(a)(1) of the OSH Act, 29 USC 651 et seq.

○ **What is the general-duty clause and why is it important?**

Each employer covered by the OSH Act has a "general duty" to provide to "each of his employees employment and a place of employment which are free from recognized hazards that are causing or are likely to cause death or serious physical harm to his employees" |29 USC 654(a)(1)|. Each employer must also comply with applicable occupational safety and health standards promulgated by the Secretary of Labor |29 USC 654(a)(2)|. The importance of the general-duty clause is the ability of OSHA inspectors to invoke it to cover any hazard not covered by an industry-specific standard.

❍ **How is the general-duty clause enforced?**

An employer can be found to be in violation of the general duty clause if it can be shown that:
a) A hazard existed.
b) The hazard was likely to cause death or serious physical harm.
c) The employer had knowledge of the hazard or should have had knowledge because the hazard had been recognized by the industry or by a reasonable person.
d) The hazard was foreseeable.
e) Workers were exposed to the hazard.

❍ **What are the three kinds of OSHA standards by mechanism of development of the standards?**

Consensus standards: Standards agreed upon by a defined organization. In the case of OSHA, the American Conference of Governmental Industrial Hygienists (ACGIH) consensus standards for threshold limit values (TLVs) were adopted in 1970 as consensus standards and renamed permissible exposure limits (PELs). Also, consensus standards were adopted in 1972 from the National Fire Prevention Association (NFPA) and the American National Standards Institute (ANSI).

Temporary emergency standards: Standards that because of an agreed-upon high risk are granted to OSHA in less than the normal development interval.

New or amended standards: Standards developed according to a standard procedure of carefully considering all available and new evidence.

❍ **What is the difference between OSHA specification standards and OSHA performance standards?**

Specification standards set out precise rules for an employer to follow to satisfy an exposure standard, although employers may request waivers ("variances") from OSHA. Most OSHS safety standards are of this type. Performance standards prescribe exposure limits but leave the means of achieving those standards up to employers. Most OSHA health standards are performance standards, which despite their flexibility do not excuse employers from willful substitution of methods of questionable efficacy.

❍ **What safety standards does OSHA require?**

OSHA standards for safety are generally grouped by occupation or hazard and include regulations relating to falls, confined spaces, lock-out/tag-out, noise, bloodborne pathogens, generic carcinogens, etc. Among the most important general safety regulations are those pertaining to hazard communication, employee training, specific limits for exposure to selected hazards, recording of occupational illnesses and injuries, and access to medical records.

❍ **What is the OSHA Hazard Communication Standard (HCS, "Haz-Com")?**

The OSHA Hazard Communication Standard (29 CFR Parts 1910, 1915, 1917, 1918, 1926, and 1928) requires employers to establish hazard communication programs to transmit information on the hazards of chemicals to their employees by means of labels on containers, material safety data sheets, and training programs. These hazard communication programs are designed to ensure all employees have the "right-to-know" the hazards and identities of the chemicals they work with, and will reduce the incidence of chemically-related occupational illnesses and injuries.

○   What does the OSHA HCS specifically require?

A written program by employers for hazard communication.
Employee training regarding hazards in the workplace.
The generation of Material Safety Data Sheets (MSDSs) by manufacturers of dangerous substances and the provision of MSDSs to the employer and, ultimately, to employees.
The legal right for employees, their representatives, and physicians to inspect the MSDSs.

○   What are the training requirements mandated by the OSHA HCS?

Under the OSHA HCS, employers must explain the OSHA requirements, specify the workplace operations that involve hazardous chemicals, explain how to read MSDSs and labeling systems for hazardous substances, point out the locations of MSDSs, give the location of hazardous-materials inventories, specify available protective measures, and describe the hazards associated with nonroutine tasks.

○   What is the hazard against which lock-out, tag-out was designed?

Officially, "hazardous energy" from the inadvertent activation of a device.

○   What is the difference between lockout (and a lockout device) and tagout (and a tagout device)?

The official OSHA definitions are as follows:

"Lockout." The placement of a lockout device on an energy isolating device, in accordance with an established procedure, ensuring that the energy isolating device and the equipment being controlled cannot be operated until the lockout device is removed.

"Lockout device." A device that utilizes a positive means such as a lock, either key or combination type, to hold an energy isolating device in the safe position and prevent the energizing of a machine or equipment. Included are blank flanges and bolted slip blinds.

"Tagout." The placement of a tagout device on an energy isolating device, in accordance with an established procedure, to indicate that the energy isolating device and the equipment being controlled may not be operated until the tagout device is removed.

"Tagout device." A prominent warning device, such as a tag and a means of attachment, which can be securely fastened to an energy isolating device in accordance with an established procedure, to indicate that the energy isolating device and the equipment being controlled may not be operated until the tagout device is removed.

O   **What is a PEL?**

PEL stands for "permissible exposure limit." In 1970, the existing 1968 ACGIH TLVs (see C.3.) were adopted in their entirety by OSHA as PELs. TLVs were (and are) not legally enforceable, but OSHA PELs are published in the Code of Federal Regulations (CFR) and are enforceable under the OSH Act. They, like TLVs, are meant to represent the level to which an employee could be exposed for 8 hours a day, 5 days a week for the duration of his or her employment without suffering adverse health effects, although these levels have not been validated scientifically and are not to be equated with proven safe levels. Instead, they serve as regulatory standards used for determining an employer's legal responsibility.

O   **What does the PEL have to do with the initiation of corrective action by an employer?**

Employers must take action when levels reach the OSHA action level, defined as ½ of the PEL.

O   **How are PELs upgraded?**

OSHA tried in 1989 to accomplish a wholesale update of the PELs but was challenged in court and lost. Since that time, OSHA has had to justify every proposed upgrade on an individual basis.

O   **Must every state abide by the OSHA PELs?**

Essentially, yes: states may substitute their own permissible exposures, but they must be at least as strict as the OSHA PELs.

O   **What does the PEL have to do with the initiation of corrective action by an employer?**

Employers must take action (e.g., medical surveillance, exposure monitoring) when levels reach the OSHA action level, defined as ½ of the PEL.

O   **To what degree could one assume that abidance by PELs will assure worker safety?**

Neither PELs nor TLVs have been scientifically validated, and evidence exists to suggest that they are in fact set too high to protect employees. Thus, a single value should never be used to make a final determination on the exposure hazards at a given worksite.

O   **What is an REL?**

REL stands for "recommended exposure limits." RELs were developed by NIOSH in its criteria documents. RELs are recommendations and not legally enforceable. They often tend to be lower than PELs and TLVs, partly because of additional investigations and partly because of the NIOSH practice of using ten-hour workdays instead of eight-hour workdays.

❍ **What is an 8-hour TWA?**

OSHA considers a work day to last eight hours. The legally enforceable OSHA 8-hour TWA is the average concentration of an airborne toxicant during an 8-hour work period. Brief periods slightly above and below this value are typical and are permitted as long as the average for the 8-hour period does not exceed the TWA.

❍ **What are C limits and STELs?**

Ceiling limits (C limits) are those levels that cannot for any reason be exceeded at any time during any part of the work day. Short-term exposure limits (STELs) are allowable 15-minute exposure levels above the TWA. There may be no more than 4 STEL periods in a work day and there must be 60 minutes between the periods. STELS must be balanced with much lower exposures during the day so that the average exposure does not exceed the TWA. STELS are not available for all substances. Both ceiling limits and STELs are legally enforceable.

❍ **What are ANSI standards?**

These standards, developed by the American National Standards Institute, are consensus standards that have been incorporated into Federal law as 29 CFR 1910.1000 (Table Z-2). As such, they are legally enforceable under the OSH Act.

❍ **What are TLVs?**

TLVs, or threshold limit values, were levels developed in 1946 by a committee of the American Conference of Governmental Industrial Hygienists (ACGIH). The TLVs were designed to "refer to airborne concentrations of substances and represent conditions under which it is believed that nearly all workers may be repeatedly exposed day after day |8 hours a day, 5 days a week, for a working lifetime| without adverse health effects." The ACGIH also warned that "because of wide variation in individual susceptibility, however, a small percentage of workers may experience discomfort from . . . concentrations below the threshold limit."

❍ **What is the meaning of the "skin" notation associated with some TLVs?**

The skin notation denotes that absorption through the skin may be significant with the specified toxicant and that respiratory protection alone may therefore be insufficient.

❍ **How have TLVs been used?**

As previously mentioned, TLVs were adopted whole cloth into the OSH Act in 1970. Since then, the ACGIH has continued to update the TLVs, which are propounded as guides only and are not legally enforceable. Exposure to less than a TLV has often been interpreted as guaranteeing safe working conditions, but as the ACGIH has stated, "The limits are not fine lines between safe and dangerous concentrations nor are they a relative index of toxicity, and should not be used by anyone untrained in the discipline of industrial hygiene." The TLVs were initially developed as a compromise between health concerns and industry costs and have not been scientifically validated.

○ **What are BEIs?**

BEIs, or biological exposure indices, were also developed by the ACGIH. They provide warning levels of biological responses to a substance or agent, or warning levels of the substance or agent or its metabolite(s) in the tissues, fluids, or exhaled air of an exposed worker. They are the biological-monitoring equivalent of TLVs for exposure monitoring. A given level from an exposed worker compared with the BEI for that exposure is of little value unless the specimen has been drawn at appropriate times relative to a worker's exposure. As with TLVs, BEIs are to be used only in conjunction with designated exposure standards or codes of practice and not as a sole method for exposure control.

○ **What are the names of the illness-and-injury records currently required by OSHA?**

a) OSHA Form 300   (Log of Work-Related Injuries and Illnesses)
b) OSHA Form 300A (Summary of Work-Related Injuries and Illnesses)
c) OSHA Form 301   (Injury and Illness Incident Report)

○ **Does the requirement to keep OSHA Forms 300, 300A, and 301 apply to all industries?**

No. Low-risk industries with certain Standard Industry Classification (SIC) codes (see http://www.osha.gov/recordkeeping/ppt1/RK1exempttable.html) are exempt, as are employers with ten or fewer employees. However, work-related incidents resulting in a fatality occurs or in the hospitalization of three or more employees must be reported regardless of industry-specific exemptions. Also, all employers selected by the Bureau of Labor and Statistics (BLS) for BLS surveys must keep these OSHA forms during the period of time covered by the survey regardless of official exemption by OSHA.

○ **Under the 200-series forms replaced by OSHA Forms 300, 300A, and 301, any aggravation of a pre-existing condition by a workplace event or exposure made a case work-related. How has that guidance changed under the new rules in effect concerning the 300-series forms?**

Aggravation of a pre-existing condition is now considered to be work-related only if the aggravation is significant.

○ **With OSHA Forms 300, 300A, and 301, nine conditions exempt an injury from being considered work-related. What are they?**

Being a member of the general public.
Symptoms arising on work premises but totally due to outside factors.
Voluntary participation in a workplace wellness program.
Preparing, eating, or drinking one's own food.
Personal tasks outside working hours.
Personal grooming, self-medication, and self-inflicted injuries.
A motor-vehicle accident in a parking lot or an access road during a commute to or from work.
A cold or flu (influenza).
Mental illness (unless the employee voluntarily presents a medical opinion to document that the employee has a mental illness that is work-related).

(See http://www.osha.gov/recordkeeping/RKside-by-side.html.)

○ **T/F: Employee medical records are the property of the employee.**

False. They usually are construed to be the property of the company.

○ **What do OSHA regulations require concerning employee access to medical records?**

OSHA standards for each category of industry require that employers grant an employee access to any of his or her medical records maintained by the employer and to any employer-maintained records on the employee's exposure to toxic substances.

○ **If an employee requests an employer to provide medical and environmental data to him or her concerning an exposure, how long does OSHA give the employer to furnish this information?**

15 days.

○ **T/F: An exposed employee can request from his or her employee records of toxic exposures of other exposed employees.**

True, if the requested data is relevant to the likelihood of exposure of the employee requesting the data.

○ **What are possible legal consequences of improper disclosure of employee medical information?**

Civil action brought by the employee on the basis of invasion of privacy.
Action of a professional licensing board based upon unauthorized disclosure of a medical confidence.

○ **OSHA standards for each type of industry except for agriculture include specifically stated requirements regarding personal protective equipment. In general, what do these standards require of employers?**

Provision, at no cost to employees, of personal protective equipment for certain hazards encountered in the industry.

○   **OSHA requirements for personal protective equipment conform to the levels of protection defined by the Environmental Protection Agency (EPA). What are these levels?**

Levels A (the highest level), B, C, and D (see http://www.ehso.com/OSHA_PPE_EPA_Levels.htm).

○   **Where is the OSHA respiratory protection standard found?**

29 CFR 1910.134 (see also http://www.ehso.com/RespProtection_Majoreq.htm).

○   **Every workplace covered by the OSH Act is subject to inspection by representatives either of OSHA or of the applicable state occupational-safety-and-health agency. What are these representatives called?**

Compliance safety and health officers (CSHOs).

○   **OSHA can levy penalties for several OSHA-defined types of violations. What are the types of violations that OSHA can find?**

Other-than-serious violations.
Serious violations.
Willful violations.
Repeated violations.
Failure to correct a repeat violation.
Falsifiying records.
Violations of posting requirements.
Assaulting or otherwise interfering with a compliance officer.

○   **For which types of OSHA violations can criminal penalties be imposed?**

Willful violation resulting in the death of an employee.
Falsifying records.
Assaulting or otherwise interfering with a compliance officer.

○   **Under the Mine Safety and Health Act of 1977 (MSHA), how frequently must each underground mine be fully inspected?**

Four times a year.

○   **What portion (Title) of what federal statute prohibits employment discrimination on the basis of race, color, religion, sex, national origin, age, and disability?**

Title VII of the Civil Rights Act of 1964.

❍   **An amendment to Title VII of the Civil Rights Act of 1964 protects workers against discrimination based on pregnancy. What is this amendment called?**

The Pregnancy Discrimination Act of 1978.

❍   **What independent federal agency administers the Civil Rights Act of 1964 as well as the Equal Pay Act of 1963, the Age Discrimination Employment Act of 1967 (ADEA), Sections 501 and 505 of the Rehabilitation Act of 1973, Titles I and V of the Americans with Disabilities Act of 1990 (ADA), and the Civil Rights Act of 1991?**

The Equal Employment Opportunity Commission, or EEOC.

❍   **T/F: According the Age Discrimination Employment Act of 1967 (ADEA), employment discrimination based upon age is determined to be unlawful for all employees over the age of 21 years.**

False. The ADEA protects employees and job applicants who are 40 years old or older.

❍   **In 1990, the ADEA was amended to forbid employers from denying benefits to older employees. What is the name of this amendment?**

The Older Workers Benefit Protection Act of 1990, or OWBPA.

❍   **What federal law provides up to 12 weeks of job-protected unpaid leave during any 12 months for the birth of an employee's child or for adoption of a child by an employee?**

The Family and Medical Leave Act of 1993 (FMLA).

❍   **For what other two major conditions can an employee request up to 12 weeks of job-protected unpaid leave during any 12-month period?**

Care for a spouse, child, or parent with a serious health condition.
A serious health condition involving the employee himself or herself.

❍   **Which section (Title) of the Americans with Disabilities Act of 1990 (ADA) applies specifically to employment?**

Title I.

❍   **The ADA requires employers to provide reasonable accommodations (that are not an undue hardship) for any qualified individual with a disability who can perform the essential functions of a job. However, there is an important exception to this provision. Name the exception.**

When a direct threat (a significant risk of substantial harm, taking into account the duration, the likelihood, the imminence, and the severity of the harm) exists, reasonable accommodation need not legally be provided.

○   **What are the three components of the definition of a disability under the ADA?**

The presence of a physical or mental impairment that substantially limits one or more major life activities.
Having a record of such an impairment.
Being regarded as having such an impairment.

○   **T/F: An employer with 18 employees would be exempt from the ADA.**

False. The original exemption was for employers with fewer than 25 employees, but within two years of passage of the act only employers with fewer than 15 employees were exempt.

○   **T/F: Drug testing, fitness for duty, medical surveillance, return to work, and impairment examinations are unaffected by the ADA.**

True.

○   **T/F: The ADA prohibits medical screening for future illness, injury, or liability.**

True.

○   **What legislation enacted in 1988 requires all federal agencies, grant recipients, and contractors to certify that they will maintain a drug-free workplace?**

The Drug Free Workplace Act of 1988.

○   **T/F: A workplace drug test is considered to be positive only after review by a medical review officer (MRO) who has graduated from an officially approved MRO course.**

False. A workplace drug test must be confirmed by a medical review officer before being considered positive, but the MRO need not have graduated from an MRO course.

○   **What is the role of the U.S. Environmental Protection Agency (EPA) in workplace health and safety?**

The EPA regulates pesticides via the Federal Insecticide, Fungicide, and Rodenticide Act (FIFRA); toxic chemicals via the Toxic Substances Control Act of 1976 (TSCA); and hazardous waste via the Resource Conservation and Recovery Act of 1976 (RCRA) and the Comprehensive Environmental Response, Compensation and Liability Act of 1980 (CERCLA). The major role of the EPA specifically for worker health and safety is in the protection of workers from pesticides by means of the EPA Worker Protection Standard (40 CFR Part 70).

ENVIRONMENTAL MEDICINE

HEAT-RELATED ILLNESS

❍ **What do you call swelling of the hands and feet in a non-acclimatized person?**

Heat edema.

❍ **What is the treatment for heat edema?**

No treatment is required.

❍ **What is "prickly heat"?**

Acute inflammation of sweat ducts secondary to blockage by macerated statum corneum. Also known as heat rash.

❍ **Is talc or baby powder used to treat "prickly heat"?**

No benefit.

❍ **How do you prevent "prickly heat"?**

Loose fitting clothing.

❍ **What is "chronic heat rash"?**

Sweat gland secondary infection with Staphlococcus Aureus following acute "prickly heat".

❍ **What is the treatment for "chronic heat rash"?**

Dicloxacillin to eradicate Staphlococcus Aureus.

❍ **What is "heat syncope"?**

Postural hypotension in and unacclimatized person in early heat exposure.

❍ **What is the treatment for "heat syncope"?**

Removal, fluids and acclimatization.

❍ **Is "heat syncope" the result of low blood volume?**

No.

○ **How do you prevent "heat syncope"?**

Slow progressive acclimatization.

○ **What are "heat cramps"?**

Involuntary muscle contractions secondary to hyptonic fluid replacment.

○ **Can "heat cramps" be treated with water rehyrdation?**

No. Electrolyte solutions are required for treatment to replace losses.

○ **What occupations are at risk for "heat cramps"?**

Unconditioned manual labor who are just starting a new job or activity.

○ **What is the underlying electrolyte imbalance in "heat cramps"?**

Hyponatremia, and to a lesser extent hypokalemia.

○ **Are salt tablets useful in the treatment of heat induced illness?**

No. Salt tablets alone are inadequate and have almost no role in heat illness treatment.

○ **What is "heat tetany"?**

Spasms of the hands and feet secondary to hyperventilation and subsequent respiratory alkalosis.

○ **What work practices are associated with "heat tetany"?**

Short periods of intense heat exposure.

○ **Do "heat cramps" accompany "heat tetany"?**

No. The underlying mechanism is different.

○ **What are the symptoms of "heat exhaustion"?**

Non specific. Nausea, weakness, fatigue, myalgia, dizziness, subjective feelings of weakness and many others.

○ **What is the diagnostic core temperature of "heat exhaustion"?**

There is not one. Temperature ranges from normal to 104°F.

O **What is the defining feature that distinguishes "heat exhaustion" from more severe heat related illness?**

Normal mental status.

O **What is the mechanism of "heat exhaustion"?**

Unacclimatized individuals exposed to a hot environment without adequate fluid and electrolyte replacement.

O **What are the laboratory findings of "heat exhaustion"?**

Hemoconcentration. All other lab values will vary based on fluid intake.

O **What are the clinical signs of "heat exhaustion"?**

Syncope, emesis, sinus tachycardia, and diaphoresis. The victims are "wet".

O **What is the treatment for "heat exhaustion"?**

Removal, rest and volume replacement.

O **What is the essential feature for "heat stroke" to be diagnosed?**

Mental status changes.

O **What is the classic heat stroke triad?**

Core temperature elevation (105°F), mental status changes, anhidrosis. *(dry)*

O **Are "heat stroke" victims wet or dry?**

Classically dry.

O **What is the core temperature requirement for "heat stroke"?**

None. 105°F was suggested by several medical societies, however no rule has been put forward.

O **What is the most sensitive neurological test for "heat stroke"?**

Gait and balance, as the cerebellum is one of the first structures effected.

O **What are the neurological signs of "heat stroke"?**

Any pattern is possible, however common associations are bizarre behavior, ataxia and hallucinations.

❍ **What is the worst temperature exposure pattern for "heat stroke"?**

Lower absolute temperature exposure for a longer period.

❍ **What is "classic heat stroke"?**

Non-exersional heat illness that occurred with early summer heat waves.

❍ **Who is most at risk for "classic heat stroke"?**

The elderly, and chronically ill (particularly cardiovascular ailments). These folks have a reduced ability to disperse heat.

❍ **What is "exertional heat stroke"?**

Increased heat production as a result of vigorous activity that overwhelms body cooling mechanisms.

❍ **Who is at risk for "exertional heat stroke"?**

Everyone, but classically younger athletic males in the summer in humid environments

❍ **Are there distinctive signs and symptoms to differentiate the types of "heat stroke"?**

No. The distinctions are of historical importance only.

❍ **What is the outcome of untreated "heat stroke"?**

Multi-organ dysfunction and death. Liver, kidney, muscle and CNS tissue necrosis is documented at temperatures of 108°F core. This temperature also interferes with the clotting cascade and electrical activity of the heart.

❍ **What are urinalysis results in "heat stroke"?**

Proteinuria, hematuria, hyaline casts are resultant from heat induced kidney damage.

❍ **Do you expect elevations of myoglobins and troponin in "heat stroke"?**

Yes. The normal markers for ischemic heart disease can result from direct myocardial insult or secondarily from hypoprofusion of the cardiac muscle.

❍ **What are coagulation test abnormalities common with "heat stroke"?**

Thrombocyotopenia, hypofibrinogenemia, and at extreme temperatures elevated markers consistent with D.I.C.

O **Should you give antipyretics to heat stroke victims?**

No.

O **What is the treatment for heat stroke?**

Removal, fluids, immediate cooling and systemic medical monitering.

O **Is cold water immersion useful in the treatment of heat related illness?**

No. The cold water results in peripheral vasoconstriction and shivering that will increase core temperatures.

O **Is room temperature water immersion useful in the treatment of heat related illness?**

No. Immersion will limit access to the patient and other modalities are more effective.

O **What is the most rapid way to cool a heat illness victim?**

Cold peritoneal lavage is the most rapid, however limited availability and invasiveness limit usefulness.

O **Where should ice packs be placed to cool victims of heal illness?**

Groin and axillae are the best locations for ice packs to cool patients without interference with other treatments.

O **At what core body temperature should cooling efforts cease?**

Core temp of 104°F.

O **What are complications of fan and water evaporative cooling?**

Shivering and vasoconstriction.

O **What medications are useful to limit shivering in a heat illness patient during cooling?**

Benzodiazepines and phenothiazines can terminate shivering to assist cooling operatons.

O **What is "overshoot hypothermia"?**

Failure to cease cooling efforts that lead to an abnormally low body temperature.

○ **What are some drugs that interfere with sweat production and increase heat susceptibility?**

Antihistamines, anticholinergics, phenothiazines, benzatropine.

○ **What is the calculation for Wet Bulb Globe Thermometer (WBGT) heat index?**

Wet x .7 + Dry x .1 +Black x .2 = index temperature

○ **What index temperature should all intense physical labor cease?**

Index temperature of 90.

○ **Are electrolyte sports drinks more effective to prevent heat related illness compared to water?**

No. Palatability is the only concern that may cause more people to choose an alternative to water.

○ **What drugs increase the body heat production and thus susceptibility to heat illness?**

Thyroid hormones, amphetamines, tricyclic antidepressants, and LSD.

○ **What drug has been shown to reduce thirst and thus increase susceptibility to hear illness?**

Haloperidol. *(Haldol)*

○ **What is the OSHA standard allowable temperature for workers?**

There is no OSHA standard related to heat.

○ **What is the TLV for heat exposure?**

This vary cumbersome calculation is little used, however many agencies have expressed interest in applying. TLV acclimatized 56.7- 11.5log10 x metabolic rate in Watts per eight hours.

○ **How long does it take for an adult worker to become acclimatized?**

For adults, the average time is 10 days, however this varies by conditioning, physical exertions and body habitus.

○ **How long does it take for children to become acclimatized?**

In general children acclimate slower than adults, however with less variability between kids. The literature supports 14 days for full acclimatizaton.

ALTITUDE-RELATED ILLNESS

○ **What is the percentage of oxygen in the atmosphere?**

Twenty-one percent. The percentage does not change with altitude.

○ **What effect does elevated altitude have on oxygen concentration?**

Although the percentage of oxygen does not change, a decreased partial pressure of total gas at altitude necessarily requires a drop in the partial pressure of oxygen at any given elevation, and thus a decreased oxygen concentration in gas.

○ **What is the definition of "High Altitude" ?**

4,900 feet – 11,500 feet above sea level.

○ **What is the definition of "Very High Altitude"?**

11,500- 18,000 feet above sea level.

○ **What is the definition of "Extreme Altitude"?**

Any elevation 18,000 feet or more above sea level.

○ **What signs and symptoms are present at "High Altitude" classically?**

Increased ventilation rate and reduced exercise tolerance in non-acclimatized persons.

○ **What is the underlying physiological dysfunction in altitude sickness?**

Reduced arterial oxygen concentration and reduced venous carbon dioxide concentration due to rapid breathing in an oxygen poor environment.

○ **What is the most important factor in determining who will develop altitude induced sickness?**

Rate of ascent. Faster climb leads to more symptoms in all individuals.

○ **What anatomic structure is principally responsible for increased respiratory rate due to the lowered PO$_2$ at altitude?**

The carotid body.

○ **During the ascent and before acclimatization, what blood findings are indicative of altitude induced illness?**

Respiratory alkalosis.

○ **What organ is responsible for balancing the elevated pH of the blood in acute altitude induced illness?**

The kidney.

○ **What drug is useful to accelerate acclimatization and reduce or remove blood markers of altitude sickness?**

Acetazolamide, which works by forcing a bicarbonate diuresis equalizing blood pH.

○ **In individuals living at altitude, what blood markers can be shown to be elevated?**

Erythropoetin, and consequently elevated red blood cell mass.

○ **What is "mountain diruesis"?**

The body's attempt to correct alkalosis from elevated respiratory rates will result in suppression of ADH secretion and increased urination or bicarbonate rich urine.

○ **What is "Altitude Induced Sleep Disorder"?**

Reduced stage III and IV sleep, and increased lighter Stage I sleep has been noted to lead to fatigue and lethargy in many altitude workers before acclimatization is completed.

○ **What is "High Altitude Syndrome"?**

Pulmonary edema, cerebral edema, retinopathy, peripheral edema and sleep problems.

○ **What are other altitude associated medical problems that are found concurrent with most altitude induced injuries?**

Increased incidence of hypothermia, frostbite, pharyngitis, traumatic injuries and UV light induced Keratitis.

○ **What is the final common pathway for treatment of all altitude induced injuries?**

Oxygen and descent.

○ **What is meant by "Acute Hypoxic Altitude Related Injury"?**

The syndrome of rapidly reduced arterial blood oxygen, respiratory alkalosis and resultant pulmonary edema found during rapid decompression of an airframe or loss of oxygen support in a high altitude worker.

○   **At what oxygen saturation level does unconsciousness occur?**

55 percent.

○   **What is the threshold for developing classical "Mountain Sickness"?**

9000 feet.

○   **What factors predispose to altitude induced illness?**

Rapid rate of ascent, old age and lung disease.

○   **Are more physically fit individuals less likely to develop altitude induced illness?**

No. Physical fitness does not appear to play any role in protection against altitude illness.

○   **What are classic symptoms of "Mountain Sickness" in workers at altitude?**

Lightheadedness, fatigue, head ache, anorexia, nausea, dyspnea and sleepiness.

○   **What is the "hallmark" of altitude illness that does not appear in persons undergoing normal acclimatization?**

Fluid retention and edema, as opposed to normal diuresis.

○   **What is the mean duration of illness symptoms in workers with acute "Mountain Sickness"?**

3 days.

○   **How do you treat workers that appear to have altitude induced sickness and are unable to rapidly descend?**

Acetazolamide, stop ascent, oxygen and analgesics.

○   **What is the underlying dysfunction in altitude induced injury that fails to respond to conservative therapy?**

Pulmonary edema. Once this occurs, the symptoms are not likely to resolve and in fact may progress to cerebral edema. This situation requires immediate descent and oxygen.

❍ **How can you hasten the recovery of moderate or severely incapacitated altitude induced workers?**

Hyperbaric oxygen therapy.

❍ **What medication has historically been utilized to treat all altitude injuries in facilities without hyperbaric treatment capability?**

Dexamethosone.

❍ **What can be done to prevent Altitude induced injury?**

Limiting ascent to 3000 feet per day, and requiring a two day layover at or above the 10,000 foot mark.

❍ **What is HACE?**

"High Altitude Cerebral Edema," a progressive neurological deterioration with altered mental status, ataxia, stupor and progression to coma.

❍ **How do you treat a HACE emergency?**

Oxygen, descent, steroids, and hyperbaric therapy.

❍ **What are unusual altitude associated illness?**

Strokes and blood clots are seen at a relatively high frequency in patients with no or few risk factors due to elevated red blood cell mass and decreased blood volume.

❍ **What is HAPE?**

High Altitude Pulmonary Edema. This is a non-cardiogenic edema that occurs due to hypoxia and alkalosis at altitude.

❍ **What are the signs and symptoms of HAPE?**

Dry cough, tachycardia, tachypnea, rales, and dyspnea on exertion. This may progress to frank edema and lead to unconsciousness.

❍ **What is the typical patient profile for HAPE?**

Young athletic males in excellent shaper prior to altitude exposure.

❍ **Are x-rays helpful in diagnosis of HAPE?**

Yes. X-ray evidence of pulmonary edema can support the decision to evacuate a worker who is suspected of having altitude-induced illness.

❍   **What is the treatment for HAPE?**

Bed rest, descent, oxygen, steroids and hyperbaric treatment.

❍   **What is altitude-induced bronchitis?**

New term for "climbers cough", cough induced by cold and dry air that is inhaled at an increased rate due to altitude exposure.

❍   **What is Monge's Disease?**

Polycythemia from excessive erythopoeiten production that leads to headache, congestion and decreased mental alertness.

❍   **What eye diseases occur at elevated altitudes?**

Altitude retinopathy (edema and swollen retinal veins) and ultraviolet keratitis (snow blindness).

❍   **Why is keratitis more common at higher altitudes?**

UV light penetrates better at altitude due to less water vapor, lessened particulate and lessened cloud cover at altitude.

❍   **What percentage of increased UV radiation occurs for each 1000 foot increase in elevation?**

Five percent increase.

❍   **What medical conditions predispose to altitude-induced injury?**

Pregnancy, Coronary ischemic conditions, sickle cells diseases and any lung damage.

❍   **In the military community, who is most at risk for altitude-induced illness?**

Unpressurized flight above 10,000 feet.

❍   **At what altitude is oxygen equipment mandated for use by the FAA?**

10,000 feet above sea level.

❍   **What is the most commonly associated incident that leads to altitude-induced illness in aviation?**

Rapid decompression.

○ **What are the effects of rapid altitude exposure in a decompression?**

Hypoxia, rapid gas (pulmonary and GI) expansion and decompression sickness.

○ **Why is breath holding dangerous during decompression?**

Rapid gas expansion must have an avenue for exit, otherwise it will result in torn lung tissue and a pnuemothorax if breath is held.

○ **What is aviation decompression sickness?**

The rapid loss of cabin pressure results in acute gas expansion in the blood, resulting in bubbles that circulate to the major organs causing damage.

○ **What is required for aviation-induced decompression sickness?**

Travel above 10,000 feet, and a loss of pressurization.

○ **What are associated symptoms of acute aviation-induced altitude sickness?**

Loss color vision, parasthesias, cold injury, and hypoxia.

○ **What medical profession breakthrough first allowed high altitude flight?**

Solid dental fillings. Damaged teeth have gas expansion and pain that limited pilot ability during World War II, until the pioneering work of Army dentists developed solid fillings.

○ **What is Otic Barotraumas?**

Rapid descent in aviation may result in low pressure in the middle ear, collapsed Eustachian Tube and eventual rupture of the tympanic membrane.

○ **What is Sinus Barotraumas?**

Rapid descent in aviation may result in low pressure in the sinus, collapse of the sinus ostia and eventual sinus rupture and blood filling. Normally this occurs only with unpressurized flight.

○ **What is the treatment for Barotrauma?**

Ascent.

○ **What is the treatment for aviation-induced decompression sickness?**

Oxygen, IV fluids and rapid transfer to hyperbaric facility.

❍   **What is the Valsalva Maneuver?**

Breathing out against a closed mouth and pinched nose to equalize the pressure in the ears and sinus for descent.

❍   **What is the best way to prevent altitude-induced illness in aviation?**

Do not fly with any signs of Eustachian or sinus dysfunction. The FAA states it this way: "Don't Fly with a URI".

UNDERSEA MEDICINE

○ **What is the number of atmospheres at sea level?**

By definition, air at sea level is 14.7 lb/in^2 or 1 atmosphere (ATA).

○ **At what depth of water is 2 ATA?**

33 feet of seawater.

○ **Where is the greatest proportionate change in pressure for unit depth?**

Near the surface. It takes progressively less change in depth for unit pressure changes near the surface.

○ **What diving pressures do most recreational scuba divers experience?**

Recreational diving is confined to pressures less than 6 ATA.

○ **What is the depth of water at 6 ATA, the maximum recreation/ normal occupational diving limit?**

165 feet of seawater.

○ **Which career fields are likely to have divers for commercial purposes?**

Natural resources gathering, maintenance, salvage, construction, rescue and sport facilities.

○ **What is Boyle's law?**

PV=K, where K is constant, P= pressure and V= volume.

○ **What happens to pressure when volume is halved?**

Using Boyle's law, it is doubled.

○ **What is Dalton's Law?**

Pt=PO2+PN2+Px. Total pressure is the sum of pressures of component gasses in a mixture.

○ **What is Henry's Law?**

%X=PxPtx100. The amount of gas dissolved in liquid is X, PX is partial pressure of gas, Pt is total atmospheric pressure. Amount of gas dissolved in liquid is proportional to pressure of gas at equilibrium.

O   **Why are Boyle's, Dalton's, and Henry's laws important in medicine?**

They explain the behavior of gas in the body at varying depths of pressure. Understanding these laws explains all the phenomena of dsybarism (depth sickness).

O   **What is the "Bends"?**

The "Bends" is a term to describe a hunched over posture assumed by dysbarically injured workers that resembled a ladies fashion trend of bending forward with a large rear hoop skirt in the 1800s. The workers are "Bent" by pain from bubbles.

O   **What is "Caisson's disease"?**

Another term for decompression sickness that originates from the relatively large amount of this type of injury seen in bridge foundation (caisson) workers.

O   **What is the treatment for "Caisson's disease"?**

Classically return to pressure environment. Today graduated recompression by hyperbaric oxygen therapy.

O   **What are the three major divisions of dive-related injury?**

Barotrauma, gas toxicity, and decompression sickness.

O   **Which is the most common dive-related illness seen in occupational divers?**

Barotrauma.

O   **What is the mechanism of Barotrauma?**

Tissue damage that results from contraction or expansion of gases in any space of the body.

O   **What is "Squeeze Barotrauma"?**

This is barotrauma that results from descent to an area of greater pressure and thus contraction of body gas.

O   **What are the primary organs of descent barotrauma?**

Hollow organs with narrow openings are at greatest risk. The ears and sinus are the most commonly injured organs. The collapse of sinus ostia or Eustachian tube, with negative pressure will result in a suction injury to the tympanic membrane or sinus lining. The final common pathway is filling with a fluid (blood) to resolve the vacuum created in the organ.

○ **What is the most common type of descent barotrauma?**

Far and away the Aural Barotrauma is most common.

○ **What are the three types of Aural Barotrauma?**

External, medial, and internal.

○ **What is the mechanism for External Barotitis?**

Obstructed ear canal leads to negative pressure chamber in the ear canal. Vacuum is generated that tissue collapse and potential tympanic membrane rupture.

○ **What is the best way to protect against External Barotitis?**

Remove cerumen and ear plugs prior to diving.

○ **What is the mechanism for Medial Barotitis?**

Blockage or closure of the Eustachian tube leads to partial vacuum development in the middle ear space. The Tympanic membrane will be sucked inward and the middle space fills with blood to compensate for pressure.

○ **What are the common symptoms of Medial Barotitis?**

Pain, vertigo, nausea and sudden loud snap in the ear that indicates ruptured ear drum.

○ **What is the best method of preventing Medial Barotitis?**

Ensuring patency of the Eustachian tube by performance of the Valsalva maneuver, and avoiding diving activity during any signs of illness.

○ **How do you perform the Valsalva maneuver?**

Hold the nose and breath out hard with the mouth closed.

○ **What is inner ear Barotitis?**

The disruption of one of the inner ear structures due to an acute change in pressure. Often rupture of Reissner's membrane or the oval window will occur with too rapid descent.

○ **What are the signs and symptoms of inner Barotitus?**

Tinnitus, vertigo, nausea, hearing loss and pain.

○ **Which is the least common of the Barotitis injuries?**

Inner ear, and this condition may be permanent.

○ **What is a "sinus squeezer"?**

A closed sinus ostia with partial vacuum formation in any sinus will result in pain and eventual sinus lining rupture to fill the void with blood on descent.

○ **What are predisposing conditions to descent injuries?**

Nasal polyps, URI, any pre-existing sinus condition.

○ **What is "Diver's mask injury"?**

A tight mask seal may lead to pressure induced injury from the vacuum generated during rapid descent. It is for this reason that masks are made to fit over the nose to allow pressure release from exhaled nasal air.

○ **Why is it important to breathe when descending?**

To insure no vacuum areas develop from low pressure in the lung, which would lead to pulmonary edema from blood rushing to the low pressure areas.

○ **What is alternobaric vertigo?**

Vertigo caused by having different pressure applied to each ear from an ear injury that leads to nausea and vertigo toward the injured ear.

○ **What organs are most affected by ascent dysbaria?**

Teeth, lungs and GI tract.

○ **What is aerogastralgia?**

Literally "air in the gut," which must come out during ascent due to gas expansion with lessened pressure. Abdominal pain and bubbling are the usual result.

○ **What is pulmonary barotrauma (PBT)?**

This is failure to breathe during rapid ascent. The lungs expand with gas until a rupture occurs and leads to pnuemothorax from over pressurization.

○ **What is a dysbaric air embolus (DAE)?**

This is when a pulmonary barotrauma results in a tear in the lung that allows gas bubbles to enter circulation. The bubbles can lodge in any organ leading to any symptom from acute paraplegia to myocardial insult.

O   **What is the most common cause of a DAE?**

Novice diver who rushes to the surface due to "low tank" pressure on gauge.

O   **What must you assume if a diver has a sudden loss of consciousness upon surfacing?**

That they have had a large DAE to the brain.

O   **What is the definitive treatment for DAE induced injury?**

Recompression in a hyperbaric chamber.

O   **What is Nitrogen Narcosis?**

Nitrogen gas at pressure has an anesthetic effect that impairs divers and limits depth to 200 feet or less.

O   **Can divers remember most accidents that occurred at depth?**

No. Nitrogen narcosis effectively eliminates memory of any events leading up to a deep depth accident.

O   **Why are divers limited to 6 ATA dives?**

The effect of nitrogen narcosis limits the ability and impairs judgment of divers below this depth.

O   **What is decompression sickness (DCS)?**

Multisystem disorder resulting from liberation of gas bubbles in low pressure environment.

O   **What is the mechanism for DCS?**

Gas equilibrium is reached at depth for blood gasses, and then a rapid rise to the surface causes off gassing of the tissues and formation of bubbles.

O   **What is the composition of most DCS bubbles?**

Nitrogen gas.

O   **What factors effect the development of DCS?**

Rate of ascent, duration of dive, maximal depth. More likely with rapid rise from a prolonged deep dive.

O   **What effects do nitrogen bubbles have in the body?**

Mechanically they block circulation in the venous or capillary system, and biochemically the bubbles may induce inflammatory cascade.

O   **What is the most likely underlying disorder if a patient has a severe brain injury from DCS?**

A patent Foramen Ovale that allows a venous bubble to enter the arterial circulation.

O   **How do nitrogen bubbles induce the development of clotting in the small circulatory pathways?**

Via direct activation of Hageman factor.

O   **What is type I DCS?**

Manifestations limited to skin, lymphatic, and musculoskeletal symptoms.

O   **What is type II DCS?**

Often this is neurological or multiorgan system involvement of the bubbles.

O   **What are the "Chocks"?**

Pulmonary manifestation of DCS that are small bubble obstruction in the lungs that can lead to very serious injury.

O   **How much of the lung tissue must be involved before symptoms develop?**

Ten percent is suggested by many authors.

O   **What are common skin manifestations of DCS?**

Pruritis, rashing, and painful localized swelling.

O   **What are the musculoskeletal symptoms of DCS?**

Joint pain, swelling, and decreased motion in any large joint.

O   **What is the cuff test of DCS?**

Pain relief in a joint when a blood pressure cuff is inflated on that area. It is thought that the cuff forces bubbles out to this area; however, they will return with symptoms when cuff is deflated.

❍   **What is "Silent DCS"?**

Bubbles in the circulation without physical manifestations. They cause no apparent clinical dysfunction.

❍   **What is the treatment of DCS?**

Low altitude transport to a recompression chamber to force bubbles back into solution and then slowly climb back to normal atmospheric pressure.

BITES AND STINGS

❍ **Approximately how many venomous snake bites occur in the US every year?**

6000-8000, although many more bites undoubtedly occur but go unreported.

❍ **Roughly how many deaths occur in the US as the result of snake bite?**

5-10 per year.

❍ **What three states have no venomous snakes?**

Maine, Alaska, and Hawaii.

❍ **What percentage of snake bites are "dry"?**

20%.

❍ **The bite of which US rattlesnake produces predominately neurologic symptoms?**

Mohave Green.

❍ **Which is the only species of sea snake to be found in continental US waters?**

Pelamis platorus.

❍ **North American rattlesnakes are members of what genus?**

Crotalidae.

❍ **Bitis aritans is also known as the:**

Puff adder.

❍ **Abdominal rigidity is associated with the bite of what arthropod?**

Black widow spider (Lacrodectus mactans).

❍ **What is the incidence of wound infection following snake bite in North America?**

The incidence is considerded to be quite low; one study reported only 1 in 33 patients who did not receive prophylactic antibiotiucs developed infection.

○ **What are the two venomous lizards found in North America?**

The gila monster (Heloderma suspectum).
The beaded lizard (Heloderma horridum).

○ **What is the genus of the only dangerous scorpion indigenpous to the continental US?**

Centeroides.

○ **What is the dangerous species of scorpion found in the United States?**

Centruroides exilicauda, the bark scorpion.

○ **To what area is the centruroides scorpion native?**

Desert southwestern United States.

○ **What is the mechanism of toxicity of the centruroides scorpion venom?**

Neurotoxins affecting sodium channel function.

○ **What is the part of the scorpion body that contains the venom glands?**

The telson.

○ **What is the "tap test" in centruroides scorpion envenomation?**

Tapping on the wound causes severe pain.

○ **What is the treatment for severe centruroides envenomation?**

Goat-derived anti-venin is available.

○ **What is the most common result of a centruroides envenomation?**

Local pain and inflammation, mild paresthesias.

○ **What group of patients are most likely to manifest severe symptoms after centruriudes envenomation?**

Children under ten years of age.

○ **What are the symptoms of severe systemic toxicity after centruroides scorpion envenomation?**

Restlessness, fasciculations, weakness, cranial nerve abnormalities, hypertension, tachycardia.

○ **What is a "dry" snakebite and how often do they occur?**

A dry bite is a bite where no envenomation occurs, about 20% of snakebites.

○ **What is the family and genus of the rattlesnake?**

Family Crotalidae, genus Crotalus.

○ **What are the five families of venomous snakes?**

Colubridae, Crotalidae, Elapidae, Hydrophidae, Viperidae.

○ **Which rattlesnake has venom that contains neurotoxins?**

The Mojave rattlesnake, Crotalus scutulatus, may cause weakness and respiratory arrest.

○ **What are the local effects of Crotalid envenomation?**

Pain, swelling, erythema, hemorrhagic bullae.

○ **What are the possible systemic effects of Crotalid envenomation?**

Nausea, vomiting, weakness, coagulopathy, thrombocytopenia, hypotension, cardiovascular collapse.

○ **What is the family and genus of the coral snake?**

Family Elapidae, genus micrurus.

○ **What are the local effects of elapid envenomation?**

Mild swelling, local paresthesias.

○ **What are the possible systemic effects of elapid envenomation?**

Nausea, vomiting, confusion, weakness, cranial nerve dysfunction, respiratory arrest.

○ **What common snakes belong to the Colubridae family?**

King snake (genus lampropeltis).

○ **What is the possible serious systemic effect of Colubridae envenomation?**

Coagulopathy.

❍ **What is the family and genus of the copperhead?**

Family Crotalidae, genus Agkistrodon.

❍ **Which family of snakes have heat sensing facial pits?**

The Crotalidae, also known as the pit vipers.

❍ **Why must victims of bites by the Mojave rattlesnake be observed longer than those bitten by other crotalids?**

The neurolotoxic effects of the venom including respiratory arrest may be delayed several hours or more.

❍ **T/F: Dead snakes cannot envenomate.**

False. Numerous cases envenomations by dead snakes have been reported.

❍ **What snake venoms were used to produce the Crotalid equine-derived antivenin?**

The Eastern diamondback rattlesnake (Crotalus adamanteus), Western diamondback rattlesnake (Crotalus atrox), Tropical rattlesnake (Crotalus durisus terrificus), and fer-de-lance (Bothrops atrox).

❍ **What snake venoms are used to make the Crofab antivenin?**

The Eastern diamondback rattlesnake (Crotalus adamanteus), Western diamondback rattlesnake (Crotalus atrox), Mojave rattlesnake (Crotalus scutulatus) and the cottonmouth (Agkistrodon piscivorus).

❍ **For which types of envenomation is the Micrurus fulvius antivenin indicated?**

Envenomation by the Eastern or Texas coral snakes (Micrurus fulvius and euryxanthus).

❍ **What delayed complication occurs commonly after equine-derived antivenin?**

Serum sickness.

❍ **What are the four families of the order Hymenoptera?**

Apidae, Bombidae, Vespidae, Formicidae.

❍ **What are the common members of each family of Hymenoptera?**

Apidae – honeybee.

Vespidae – wasps, hornets, yellow jackets.
Bombidae – bumblebees.
Formicidae – ants.

❍ **Which member of the hymenoptera order dies after stinging its victim only once?**

The honeybee.

❍ **What phylum contains the jellyfish?**

Cnidaria.

❍ **What is the name for the stinging organs on the jellyfish?**

Nematocysts.

❍ **How do nematocysts function in envenomation?**

The nematocysts fire a barb which carries venom and penetrates the victim's skin.

❍ **What is the common and scientific name for the most toxic Australian jellyfish?**

The box jellyfish, Chironex fleckeri.

❍ **What are the most common symptoms of a jellyfish sting?**

Local pain, burning, rash, pruritis.

❍ **What is the treatment for severe box jellyfish envenomation?**

Treatment with antivenin.

❍ **What is the result of severe box jellyfish envenomation?**

Acute cardiovascular collapse.

❍ **What are "tentacle tracks"?**

Linear areas of inflammation along the range of contact with a stinging jellyfish.

❍ **Why should saltwater be used to irrigate a jellyfish sting?**

Freshwater may cause the discharge of nematocysts.

❍ **What substance may be used to disarm nematocysts in a victim?**

Vinegar for most Cnidarian stings.

○ **For which Cnidarian envenomations should baking soda be used to disarm nematocysts?**

American sea nettle, little mauve stinger jellyfish, and hair "lion's mane" jellyfish- these may be worsened by vinegar.

○ **To what family and genus do lionfish belong?**

Scorpaenidae pterosis.

○ **How do the Scorpaenidae envenomate?**

They have spines on the fins that can deliver venom.

○ **What are the local effects of Scorpenidae envenomation?**

Severe pain, edema, erythema, infection, rarely neurologic symptoms.

○ **Why are Scorpaenidae envenomations particularly at risk for infection?**

The integumentary layer of the spine may be retained in the victim's skin.

○ **What is the treatment for Scorpenidae envenomation?**

Hot water to the affected area may inactivate the toxin and relieve the pain.

○ **What life-threatening symptoms may occur after stonefish envenomation?**

Hypotension, arrhythmias, pulmonary edema, myocardial infarction.

○ **What is the genus of the black widow spider?**

Lactrodectus.

○ **What serious medical conditions may be mimicked by lactrodectus envenomation?**

Myocardial infarction and peritonitis.

○ **What are the symptoms produced by lactrodectus envenomation?**

Painful muscle cramps, hypertension, tachycardia, nausea and vomiting, regional diaphoresis

○ **What does the term "necrotizing arachnidism" refer to?**

Spider bites which develop into slow-healing necrotic ulcers. These bites are usually attributed to the brown recluse but may be caused by several different types of spiders.

O   **What is the active ingredient in Loxosceles reculsa venom?**

The brown recluse venom contains a number of active compounds including sphingomyelinase D, which is a chemotactic factor for neutrophils.

O   **What is the genus of the "jumping spider"?**

Phidippus.

O   **Name two North American spiders other than the brown recluse that are associated with necrotic lesions.**

Phidippus species and the hobo spider.

O   **What potentially fatal complications may occur after brown recluse envenomation?**

Hemolysis and disseminated intravascular coagulation.

O   **What systemic symptoms may occur after brown recluse envenomation?**

Fever, malaise, nausea, myalgias.

O   **T/F: North American tarantulas do not envenomate.**

False. The North American taranulas do have weak venom but rarely causes any significant effects other than pain at the bite site.

O   **What is the treatment for the seriously ill lactrodectus mactans bite victim?**

Antivenin.

O   **From what animal is the lactrodectus mactans antivenin derived?**

The horse.

O   **What drug has been advocated for use in brown recluse envenomations and why?**

Dapsone, because it inhibits neutrophil chemotaxis.

O   **What treatment has been proven to inhibit the development of necrotic lesions after brown recluse envenomation in clinical trials?**

None.

❍   **What complications may occur following black widow envenomation during pregnancy?**

Preterm labor or spontaneous abortion.

❍   **What is the usual dose of lactrodectus mactans antivenin?**

One vial.

❍   **T/F: A positive skin test prior to the administration of equine-derived antivenin is an absolute contraindication to subsequent antivenin use.**

False. Patients with severe illness who need antivenin may be pretreated with histamine blockers and given the antivenin slowly with epinephrine if needed.

❍   **What skeletal muscle relaxer is commonly utilized in black widow envenomations?**

Methocarbamol.

COLD-RELATED MEDICAL PROBLEMS

❍ **To what disorder did Hannibal loose 23,000 troops to in a single year?**

Hypothermia

❍ **What was the treatment of Frostbite prior to 1950?**

Rubbing the effected limb with snow.

❍ **What are predisposing physical factors to cold injury?**

Humidity, wind, altitude, poor clothing and risk taking behavior.

❍ **What is "Contact Frostbite"?**

Instantaneous tissue damage as a result of skin contact with super cooled objects.

❍ **Why is humidity an important factor in cold injury?**

Low humidity leads to increased evaporative cooling from body surface, and increased heat loss.

❍ **Why is wet snow more injurious than dry hardened ice?**

The free water contact acts to conduct heat away from the skin, hastening the temperature decline.

❍ **Why is elevated altitude predisposing to cold injury?**

High altitude travel leads to dehydration, hypoxia and fatigue that contribute to severity and incidence of cold injuries.

❍ **What is the most avoidable cause of cold injury?**

Inadequate clothing wear.

❍ **Why are tight fitting clothing actually worse for cold injury?**

Tight clothing result in circulatory constriction when limbs become edematous due to initial cold injury.

O   **What percent of body heat is lost through the head and neck?**

80%.

O   **What is the most commonly forgotten portion of clothing that offers the greatest protection from heat loss?**

A coverall type hat.

O   **What is the best protection against cold related injuries?**

Changing out of wet clothing if possible.

O   **What device reduced the loss of British troops by 20,000 during WWI?**

Mandatory changing and drying of socks.

O   **What medical conditions predispose to cold induced injury?**

Any condition that limits circulation, such as diabetes, arteritis, hypovoemia, and previous cold injury.

O   **What risk group accounts for the most cold related illness in the United States?**

Alcoholics and psychiatric patients.

O   **Why do alcoholics have a propensity for cold injury?**

Alcohol impairs judgment and ability to seek shelter and judge the duration and extent of cold exposure. Alcohol also directly effects vascular tone resulting in increased heat loss.

O   **How does alcohol effect vascular tone and thus susceptibility to cold injury?**

Alcohol functions as a peripheral vasodilator.

O   **What other lifestyle choice compounds alcoholics' propensity for cold injury?**

Smoking.

O   **Which racial group is most at risk for cold induced injury?**

Dark skinned persons of warmer climate regions.

O   **What is "Chillblains"?**

Painful, inflammatory lesions on the skin of exposed areas.

O   **What causes "Chillblains"?**

Intermittant exposure to wet, non freezing environments by and unprotected individual.

O   **What body areas are most effected by "Chillblains"?**

Hands, ear lobes, and feet.

O   **What do the skin lesions of "Chillblains" look like?**

Unfortunately, they are of many types. Erythema, edema, cyanosis, plaques, nodules, ulcers and even bulla are described in the literature.

O   **How long after cold exposure will skin lesions develop?**

12 hours.

O   **What is the most likely patient complaint in "Chillblains"?**

Painful parathesias, and occasional pruritis.

O   **Who is at the greatest risk of "Chillblains"?**

Females who also have Reynaud's phenomena are the most commonly affected as a group.

O   **Is the skin frozen during "Chillblains"?**

No.

O   **What is "Trench Foot"?**

Foot injury from standing too long in the cold during WWII.

O   **What is "Immersion Foot"?**

A severe variant of cold injury caused by the prolonged limb immersion in cold water.

O   **What is the underlying pathology of "Trench Foot" and "Immersion Foot"?**

Prolonged cooling in a wet environment that damages peripheral nerves.

O   **How does "Trench Foot" present?**

Early tingling that turns to numbness and eventually complete anesthesia of the foot with associated motor loss.

❍   **Is there a palpable pulse in "Trench Foot"?**

No.

❍   **What symptoms does the patient have upon rewarming of "Trench Foot"?**

Burning pain and sensitivity. Often parts of the limb will remain anesthetic, while others will appear to have hypersensitivity to all stimuli.

❍   **What do you call the healing phase of blood return and pain in "Trench Foot"?**

Hyperemic phase.

❍   **What is the most common long term outcome of "Trench Foot"?**

Cold sensitivity.

❍   **What is the treatment for "Trench Foot"?**

Slow re-warming, bandaging and elevation. Some authorities recommend nifedipine, however there is controversy surrounding medication trials in this condition.

❍   **What is the "Hunters response"?**

Cyclical cutaneous vasodilatation and vasoconstriction in very cold environments.

❍   **What happens to the "Hunter response" through acclimatization?**

The time between cycles of vasodilatation, thus warming get progressively shorter on the skin.

❍   **What event stops the "Hunter Response", and marks the beginning of cutaneous damage?**

Depressed core body temperature.

❍   **What is phase 1 frostbite?**

Irreversible tissue damage that occurs when the skin reaches temperature below 32°F, the freezing point.

❍   **What is the characteristic of "Phase 1" frostbite?**

The formation of Ice Crystals intercellularly.

❍   **What electrolyte abnormalities are seen with "Phase 1" frostbite?**

Local NaCl concentrations have been shown to increase by 10 times normal values intracellularly.

❍ **What effect do ice crystals have other than damage due to physical size and tissue displacement?**

Crystals exert an osmotic tension that draws fluid out of the cells, leading to cellular dehydration and death.

❍ **Is warming and freezing cycles protective for Frostbite?**

Unfortunately, this common practice of short "warming" breaks for severe weather exposed persons leads to increased damage due to repetitive freeze and thaw cycles.

❍ **What is "Phase 2" Frostbite?**

Phase 2 is when reperfusion occurs to affected areas resulting in edema and rewarming.

❍ **Why is "Phase 2" Frostbite harmful?**

The reperfusion occurs through damaged capillaries, resulting in white blood cell recruitment, activation of enzymes and activation of the arachadonic acid cycle.

❍ **What is the end result of "Phase 2" Frostbite?**

Vasoconstriction separates the dead damaged tissue from the healthy tissue.

❍ **What is "Frostnip"?**

A superficial freeze injury without ice crystal formation, and absence of tissue loss.

❍ **What is the hallmark of "Frostnip"?**

Tissue and functional loss do not occur following rewarming.

❍ **What is "First Degree" Frostbite?**

Erythema, partial skin freezing, and desquamation.

❍ **What is the most common patient complaints in "First Degree" Frostbite?**

Stinging and burning of the skin surface.

❍ **What is "Second Degree" Frostbite?**

Full thickness skin freezing, edema and blister formation.

O   **What is the end result of "Second Degree" Frostbite?**

Hard eschars over the affected area.

O   **What is "Third Degree" Frostbite?**

Full thickness freezing with damage that extends to the subdermal layers. Hemorrhagic blisters and blue grey skin discoloration are common.

O   **What is the "Block of Wood" sign of "Third Degree" Frostbite?**

Patients will complain of complete anesthesia and loss of muscular tone of the effected limb, only to have intense burning and pain upon rewarming.

O   **What is the hallmark of "Third Degree" Frostbite?**

Nerve involvement that leads to loss of motor function.

O   **What is the characteristic of "Fourth Degree" Frostbite?**

Extension of the freeze injury to include the muscle, bone and tendons.

O   **What is the skin lesion of "Fourth Degree" Frostbite?**

The skin appears cyanotic, and will eventually turn to bloody blisters and eshcars. Deep aching pain is common upon rewarming.

O   **What is the prognosis of "Fourth Degree" Frostbite?**

Extremely poor. Most of this tissue is dead, and becomes a risk for gangrene and other systemic infections. Large debridement is the norm.

O   **What is the treatment of all types of Frostbite in the Emergency Room?**

Rapid rewarming in a heated circulating bath of 104°F. Expect pain, tissue swelling and continued blistering during this treatment.

O   **Does Frostbite require antibiotic coverage?**

Most sources say that for second degree and above, all patients should be covered against normal skin flora that can thrive in the newly macerated tissues.

O   **Does Frostbite require a tetanus shot?**

Yes. Frostbite is considered a dirty wound.

O **Does Frostbite require emergent surgical treatment?**

No! It is impossible to define the border of damaged tissue for several hours to days after rewarming, and early surgery is associated with higher rates of morbidity and mortality.

O **What is the aftermath of severe Frostbite for the patient?**

Permanent sensitivity to cold, pain, tingling, and hyperhidrosis.

O **What is the core temperature required to diagnose Hypothermia?**

The definition requires a core temperature of less than 95°F.

O **Name the ways in which the body can loose heat.**

Conduction, Convection, radiation and evaporation.

O **Why are neonates especially sensitive to Hypothermia?**

Large surface to total volume ration results in large heat losses.

O **What structure controls thermal homeostasis in man?**

The hypothalamous.

O **What is the most important body response to combat cold?**

Behavior change. Putting on clothing and seeking shelter are far more effective than shivering or vasoconstriction.

O **What is "Non-shivering thermogenesis"?**

Increased output of thyroid and adrenal hormones that increases body temperature through metabolism.

O **What are the "metabolic causes" of Hypothermia?**

Hypothyroidism, Hypoadrenalism, Hypopituitartism and hypothalamic disfunction.

O **What is "mild" Hypothermia?**

A body temperature of between 90 and 95°F, where the body is able to physiologically adjust and produce heat. Cardiac output rises, shivering occurs and blood pressure increases.

○ **What is the "Slowing" stage of Hypothermia?**

At temperatures less than 90°F the body cannot keep up with the ongoing heat loss and there is a progressive slowing of functions. This is especially detrimental as it impairs ability to seek shelter. Blood pressure and cardiac output begin to fall.

○ **At what temperature does shivering cease?**

Shivering ceases at 86°F.

○ **What is the characteristic EKG change of Hypothermia?**

The J wave.

○ **What is the cardiac rhythm sequence in Hypothermia?**

Sinus to atrial fibrillation with slow ventricular response, ventricular fibrillation, and finally asystole.

○ **What happens to the oxyhemoglobin dissociation curve with Hypothermia?**

Shift to the left. Impairs oxygen delivery to the tissues.

○ **What is "Cold Diuresis"?**

Cold induced loss of renal urine concentrating ability that leads to significant volume losses.

○ **Is cold exposure required for Hypothermia?**

No. A significant number occur in the summer among elderly and young children who do not have the ability to maintain core body temperature.

○ **Why is rapid whole body rewarming lethal?**

This induces peripheral vasodilation and shunting of colder blood to the core where it may lead to cold induced lethal heart rhythms.

○ **What is "Warming induced acidosis"?**

The return of blood flow from lactic acidotic muscles that have been hypoprofused in hypothermia will result in a large acid return to the central cicurlation.

○ **How do you rewarm hypothermic patients?**

Very slowly. All attempts at rapid rewarming can be fatal. This is the reverse of the frostbite doctrine which calls for rapid rewarming.

ENVIRONMENTAL DISASTERS

○ **What substance was the cause of 4000 deaths in London in 1952?**

— Smog (Sulfur dioxide). SO_2

○ **What substance caused the deaths of over 500 people in a train tunnel in Salerno, Italy in 1944?**

Carbon monoxide.

○ **What substances were implicated in 125 deaths during the Cleveland Clinic fire of 1929?**

Carbon monoxide, cyanide and nitrogen dioxide.

○ **What substance was released from Lake Nyos in 1986 and killed >1700 people and thousands of animals?**

Carbon dioxide.

○ **What substance injured 200,000 people and killed >2000 people in Bhopal, India in 1984?**

Methyl isocyanate.

○ **What is "Ginger Jake paralysis", "Jake Leg" or Jake walk"?**

In 1930, TOCP was substituted for castor oil in a "medical supplement" named Jamaican Ginger. Jamaican Ginger contained ethanol but was not subject to prohibition because of its supplement status. Drinkers of Jamaican Ginger developed a neuropathy that had incomplete resolution with the discontinuation of Jamaican Ginger ingestion.

○ **What enzyme does TOCP inhibit to cause "Ginger Jake paralysis"?**

Neuropathy target esterase (NTE).

○ **What illness has been associated with the sale of tryptophan that was produced in a particular factory in Asia?**

The eosinophilia-myalgia syndrome.

○ **What substance was the cause of Epping jaundice?**

279

Methylenedianiline.

○ **What is "Yusho" (rice oil disease)?**

In 1968 in Japan, rice oil was accidentally contaminated with polychlorinated biphenyls and ingested by thousands of people leading to sensory neuropathy.

○ **What disease was associated with hexachlorobenzene exposure in Turkey, 1956?**

4000 cases of porphyria cutanea tarda.

○ **What food contaminant was associated with 40,000 deaths in Aquitania, France in 994?**

Ergots (claviceps purpurea).

○ **Ingestion of what substance is associated with Itai-Itai ("ouch-ouch) disease in Japan?**

Cadmium.

○ **What substance caused 400 deaths from ingestion of grain in Iraq, 1971?**

Methyl mercury.

○ **What substance is associated with "toxic oil syndrome" in greater than 19,000 people in Spain, 1981?**

Rape seed oil with 2% aniline.

○ **What are the signs/ symptoms of "toxic oil syndrome"?**

Pulmonary hypertension, pneumonitis, eosinophilia, and scleroderma-like skin changes.

○ **What substance was responsible for the shyness and mental status changes seen in hat manufacturers in 1800s New Jersey?**

Mercury (mercurous nitrate).

○ **What substance contaminated bread and wine and caused 40,000 cases of polyneuropathy in France, 1828?**

Arsenious acid.

○   **What substance caused the deaths of 498 people in the Coconut Grove nightclub in Boston, 1948?**

Carbon monoxide and cyanide.

○   **What substance is associated with producing headache, gastrointestinal symptoms, seizures, death and neuronal loss in Prince Edward Island, 1987?**

Domoic acid.

○   **What substance was associated with 1000 symptomatic cases after ingestion of watermelons in Oregon and California in 1985?**

Aldicarb-contaminated watermelons.

○   **What substance is associated with the onset of 192 seizures after ingestion of sugar in Pakistan, 1984?**

Endrin, a pesticide.

○   **What meperidine analog caused parkinsonism in San Jose, 1982?**

MPTP (1-methyl-4-phenyl-1,2,3,6-tetrahydropyridine).

○   **What substance resulted in 911 suicidal/homicidal deaths in Jonestown, Guyana in 1978?**

Cyanide.

○   **What substance was leaked from a punctured tanker car and produced 8 deaths and 130 injured in Youngstown, Florida in 1978?**

Chlorine.

○   **What cancer was associated with vinyl chloride use in PVC polymerization in Louisville, Kentucky?**

Hepatic angiosarcoma.

○   **What substance was released into Minamata Bay, Japan in the 1950s?**

Mercury.

○   **What symptoms were found in children living around Minamata Bay?**

Brain damage, developmental delay, ocular and hearing deficits, and congenital defects.

❍   **What substance was used by several beer producers and produced cardiomyopathy?**

Cobalt.

❍   **What substance was a contaminant in sugar used in beer production in Staffordshire, England in 1900?**

Arsenic.

❍   **What substance was associated with scrotal cancer in chimney sweeps in England, 1700s?**

Polycyclic aromatic hydrocarbons (PAHs).

❍   **What led to "phossy jaw" in matchmakers in the mid 1800s?**

Exposure to white phosphorous.

❍   **What abnormality is associated with worker exposure to 1,2-Dibromo-chloropropane (DBCP)?**

Decrease in sperm motility and number.

❍   **What skin abnormality was associated with release of dioxin in Seveso, Italy?**

Chloracne.

❍   **What substance is associated with the death of hundreds of miles of wildlife in the Danube River, Romania, 2000?**

Cyanide released into the river.

❍   **What substance is associated with an increase in bone-cancer in watch dial-painters in Orange, New Jersey in the 1910s and 1920s?**

Radium.

❍   **What substance is associated with the "gasping syndrome"?**

Benzyl alcohol used in intravenous flushes led to acidosis, gasping and death of several neonates in 1981.

❍   **Contamination of acetaminophen with what substance led to the deaths of 88 children in Haiti, 1996?**

Diethylene glycol.

○ **What substance was associated with neurotoxicity in Stalinon users in France, 1954?**

Triethyltin.

○ **What substance was found in the blood of children who lived near a smelter in Kellogg, Idaho in 1975?**

98% of 1-9 year old children had blood lead concentrations greater than 40 mcg/dL.

○ **What substance contaminated cooking oil in Morocco in 1959?**

Triorthocresylphosphate (TOCP) in turbojet lubricant contaminated the cooking oil.

○ **What substance was found in "moonshine" produced in a Jackson, Michigan prison in 1979?**

Methanol.

WATER POLLUTION

○ **What percentage of the earth's water supply is in the form of fresh water?**

3 percent.

○ **What percent of the freshwater is in the form of groundwater?**

1 percent.

○ **What percentage of water that reaches the earth surface (precipitation) evaporates back into the atmosphere?**

70 percent.

○ **What percent of the precipitation becomes groundwater?**

10 percent of precipitation.

○ **Chemicals move between media in a dynamic nature. Give an example.**

Air and water, soil and water, or soil and air.

○ **Define water pollution.**

Any physical, biological or chemical alteration in water quality that adversely affects living organisms or renders the water unsuitable for consumption.

○ **When water in the atmosphere is collected, it is referred to as?**

Protected runoff.

○ **What air pollutant contributes to acid rain?**

Sulfur oxides.

○ **In water pollution terminology, what is sorption?**

The adhesion of substance to the surface of a solid.

○ **What is aeration?**

The process of bubbling air through a solution to enhance evaporation.

○ **What is the term alluvial?**

A term used to describe despots of sand or silt near stream beds.

○ **What is the biological oxygen demand?**

The oxygen use requirement of microorganisms in water rich with organic material.

○ **What is the term eutrophication refer to?**

The process of enrichment of water by nutrients.

○ **How can water pollution contribute to eutrophication?**

Substances moving from point or area sources may contribute a excess of nutrients, which may enhance aging of the water mass.

○ **What is flocculation?**

The process of agglomeration of finely divided particles into larger particles.

○ **How is groundwater defined?**

Precipitation that does not evaporate and is usually found underground percolating through in permeable rock, sand or gravel.

○ **What is surface water?**

Water on the surface of the ground that is exposed to the atmosphere.

○ **What is the term infiltration mean in water toxicology?**

The movement of flow from the surface downward into solid material.

○ **Describe the hydrologic cycle (water cycle).**

The cycle of water movement from the atmosphere to the earth and ultimately back into the atmosphere.

○ **What is leaching?**

The process by which soluble substances (nutrients and pollutants) in the soil are washed down into a lower layer of soil or dissipated.

○ **What is the maximum contaminant level (MCL)?**

The maximum permissible concentration of a contaminant in water that is being delivered to a public water system that is protective of health effects.

○ **What is the maximum contaminant level goal (MCLG)?**

An unenforceable concentration of a contaminant in water that is being delivered to a public water system that is protective of health effects.

○ **What is a point source of water pollution?**

Discharge from a defined point such as a sewer pipe effluent.

○ **What is an example of area or "non-point" water pollution?**

Fertilizer run off from an agricultural area. *(pollution that comes from many different sources)*

○ **What is potable water?**

Drinking water.

○ **What is a watershed?**

The area of land that contributes to the surface run off to a common drainage system.

○ **What large eastern United States cities, utilize water form protected watersheds?**

Boston and New York.

○ **How can VOC's enter homes from groundwater, without being the drinking water?**

High vapor pressure may evaporate out of groundwater through the vadose zone into the air around and in the home, similar to radon.

○ **MCL's are divided into "primary" and "secondary". What are primary MCL's?**

These refer to chemicals, which may pose and adverse health effect.

○ **What are secondary MCL's?**

Those that have undesirable aesthetic effects in taste, odor, or appearance of water.

○ **What is the MCL for arsenic?**

0.05 mg/L.

❍   **What is the MCL for benzene?**

0.005 mg/L.

❍   **What is the MCL for carbon tetrachloride?**

0.005 mg/L.

❍   **What is the MCL for cyanide?**

0.2 mg/L.

❍   **What is the MCL for aldicarb?**

0.007 mg/L.

❍   **What is the MCL for diquat?**

0.02 mg/L.

❍   **What is the MCL for glyphosate?**

0.7 mg/L.

❍   **What is the MCL for lindane?**

0.0002 mg/L.

❍   **What is the MCL for mercury?**

0.002 mg/L.

❍   **What is the MCL for nitrate?**

10 mg/L.

❍   **What is the MCL for nitrite?**

1 mg/L.

❍   **What is the MCL for radon?**

300 pCi/L.

❍   **What is the MCL for tetrachlorethylene?**

0.005 mg/L.

O   **What is the MCL for trichloroethylene?**

0.005 mg/L.

O   **What is the MCL for vinyl chloride?**

0.002 mg/L.

O   **What was the first legislative act aimed at improving water quality?**

The Rivers and Harbors Act of 1899.

O   **What was the first major clean water legislative act aimed at improving water quality in the United States?**

The Federal Water Pollution Control Act (FWPCA) of 1948.

O   **What was the FWPCA renamed?**

Clean Water Act.

O   **When was the Clean Water Act passed?**

1972.

O   **What was the intent of the Clean Water Act?**

To eliminate the discharge of pollutants into navigable waters and to make the waters swimmable and fishable.

O   **How does the Safe Drinking Water Act (SDWA) differ from the Clean Water Act?**

The SDWA applies primarily to water delivered to homeowners thought municipal water systems. It also protects aquifers and groundwater quality.

O   **What is the reference dose (RfD)?**

A calculation of daily oral exposure to the human population that is likely without appreciable risk of deleterious effects over a lifetime.

O   **What is the RfD of arsenic?**

None.

○   **What is the RfD for mercury?**

0.003 mg/kg/day.

○   **What is the RfD for glyphosate?**

mg/kg/day.

○   **What is the typical water intake per day in a human?**

2500 ml/day.

○   **What rule-of-thumb is a fair estimate of exposure to substances from all water sources.**

Double the daily drinking water intake for a total of 2-5 liters per day.

○   **Regarding VOC's, a 10-minute shower is equivalent to drinking how much water?**

1.4 liters of water.

○   **In addition to a shower VOC exposure, what percent comes from the bathroom?**

One third of daily exposure occurs in the bathroom (in addition to the shower).

○   **What is an aerosol?**

Liquid droplets or solid particles dispersed in air that is fine enough particle size (0.01 to 100 micrometers) to remain so dispersed for a period of time.

○   **What is a vapor?**

A vapor is the gaseous state of any material that would, under normal temperatures and pressures (NTP – 1 atm, 25°C), be a solid or a liquid.

○   **What is an aerosol?**

An Aerosol is a suspension of liquid or solid particles in the air. Particles diameters usually fall in the range: $0.01\mu \leq$ |particle diameter| $\leq 100\mu$.

○   **What is a mist?**

A Mist is an aerosol suspension of liquid particles in the air, Usually formed either by condensation directly from the vapor or by some mechanical process. Typical mist droplets have aerodynamic diameters in the range: $40\ \mu m \leq$ |aerodynamic diameter| $\leq 400\ \mu m$.

○   **What is non-point source pollution?**

Non-point source (NPS) pollution, unlike pollution from industrial and sewage treatment plants, comes from many diffuse sources.

○   **What is turbidity in water assessment?**

It is the measure of the relative cloudiness of water. Turbidity is caused by suspended solid matter scattering light as it passes through water.

○   **What is "hard water"?**

Water hardness is a historical term expressing the total concentration of cations, specifically calcium ($Ca2+$), magnesium ($Mg2+$), iron ($Fe2+$) and manganese ($Mn2+$) in water. Hardness, however, refers primarily to the amount of calcium and magnesium ions present.

○   **What is stream hardness?**

A stream's hardness reflects the geology of the catchment area and provides a measure of the influence of human activity in a watershed. For instance, acid mine drainage often results in the addition of iron ($Fe2+$) into a stream.

○   **What are oligotrophic waters?**

Waters with calcium levels of 10 ppm or less are usually oligotrophic, supporting only sparse plant and animal life.

○   **What are eutrophic waters?**

Eutrophic waters typically have calcium levels above 25 ppm.

○   **What is the term used to describe when the total hardness of water exceeds the total alkalinity?**

This is referred to as "no carbonate hardness" and indicates the presence of chloride and sulfate ions.

○   **What is the Biological oxygen demand (BOD)?**

BOD is the measure of the amount of oxygen consumed by microorganisms in aerobic oxidation of organic material. Unpolluted natural waters will have a BOD of 5 mg/L or less.

○   **Nitrogen in the forms of ammonia and nitrates functions as a plant nutrient, which initiates what process?**

Eutrophication.

❍ **What is the main source of <u>human-influenced</u> <u>nitrate</u> addition to streams?**

Sewage.

❍ **What is the United States largest water pollution source?**

Non-point sources.

OUTDOOR AIR POLLUTION

○ **What are Hazardous Air Pollutants (HAPs)?**

Those pollutants that are known or suspected to cause cancer or other serious health effects, such as reproductive effects or birth defects, or adverse environmental effects.

○ **How many HAPs are there defined in the Clean Air Act?**

188.

○ **What is a thermal inversion?**

Temperature changes that, when associated with certain air patterns, result in air, and thus pollutants being trapped over an area.

○ **What is smog?**

Photochemical pollution that result from the effect of sunlight on oxides in the atmosphere.

○ **What oxides are components of smog?**

Oxides of nitrogen and sulfur.

○ **What is ozone?**

O_3.

○ **What other substances are major produces of photochemical air pollution?**

Ozone.

○ **What is the primary target organ for photochemical air pollution?**

Respiratory tract.

○ **What are other tissues that may be affected by air pollution?**

Mucous membranes of the eyes, lead exposure from leaded gasoline in some countries.

○ **What physical or chemical properties are important in depth of penetration of the respiratory tract?**

Solubility, size, minute ventilation of host.

❍ **Where are large particle filtered?**

Upper respiratory tract.

❍ **What is a respirable particle?**

One that enters with the title volume and exits without remaining in the lung.

❍ **What is the typical size of a respirable particle?**

< 1 micron.

❍ **What is the PM10?**

Particles that measure greater than 10 microns in diameter.

❍ **What is PM2.5?**

Particles that measure greater than 2.5 microns in diameter.

❍ **What is acid deposition?**

It is the process by which acidic particles, gases, and precipitation leave the atmosphere. More commonly referred to as acid rain, acid deposition has two components: wet and dry deposition.

❍ **What is "Acid rain"?**

It is a broad term describing acid rain, snow, fog, and particles.

❍ **What causes acid rain?**

Sulfur dioxide and nitrogen oxides released from several sources including power plants, vehicles, and other sources cause acid rain.

❍ **What are some potential effects of acid rain?**

It may harm certain plants, animals, and fish, and can erodes building surfaces.

❍ **How is acid rain better described?**

A more precise term is acid deposition, which has two parts: wet and dry.

❍ **What is wet deposition?**

Wet deposition refers to acidic rain, fog, and snow.

❍ **What is dry deposition?**

Dry deposition refers to acidic gases and particles.

❍ **The ozone layer is a protective barrier located in which atmospheric layer?**

Stratosphere.

❍ **How far above the earths surface is the stratosphere?**

Approximately 22 miles above the Earth's surface.

❍ **How does the ozone layer protect?**

This layer protects us from the sun's harmful ultraviolet radiation.

❍ **What substances are allegedly harming the ozone layer?**

(CFCs)   *CFCs, BFCs, NO₂*

Chlorofluorocarbons, halons, and methyl chloroform.

❍ **What cause haze in our atmosphere?**

Haze is caused when sunlight encounters, and reflects off of tiny particles in the air.

❍ **How much of the atmospheric acidity falls back to earth?**

About half.

❍ **What are the two major components of acid rain?**

Sulfur dioxide (SO2) and nitrogen oxides (NO_x) are the primary causes.

❍ **In the US, what portion of SO_2 comes from coal powered electrical generating units?**

About 2/3 of all SO_2.

❍ **In the US, what portion of NO_x comes from coal powered electrical generating units?**

About 1/4 of all NO_x comes from electric power generation that relies on burning fossil fuels like coal.

❍ **What measure is used to determine the acidity of rain?**

pH.

O   **What is the normal pH of rainwater?**

Normal rain is slightly acidic because carbon dioxide dissolves into it, so it has a pH of about 5.5.

O   **What is the pH of acid rain?**

Most acidic rain falling in the US in the year 2000 had a pH of about 4.3.

O   **What EPA program monitors wet deposition acid rain?**

The National Atmospheric Deposition Program measures wet deposition.

O   **What EPA program measures dry deposition acid rain?**

The Clean Air Status and Trends Network (CASTNET) measures dry deposition.

O   **When was the Clean Air Act (CAA) originally enacted?**

1963.

O   **What is one of the major aspects of the CAA?**

To mandate and establish standards for airborne pollution.

O   **What is this process called?**

The National Ambient Air Quality Standards (NAAQS).

O   **The NAAQS were developed to define allowable airborne concentrations of substances referred to as?**

Criteria Pollutants.

O   **There are also secondary standards, what are they enacted to accomplish?**

To provide a measure of protection to plants and animals.

O   **The CAA provides areas with one of three designations. What are they?**

Attainment, Non-attainment, or Unclassifiable within he standards.

O   **Name two criteria pollutants?**

Criteria Pollutants
Lead, CO, NO$_2$, SO$_2$, O$_3$, PM

Carbon monoxide, lead.

O **Name two more criteria pollutants?**

Nitrogen dioxide, ozone.

O **Name another two criteria pollutants?**

Particulates and sulfur dioxide.

O **The 1990 amendments to the CAA extended the scope to include?**

Acid rain and ozone depletion.

O **What is the NAAQS for ozone?**

0.12 ppm (maximum daily 1-hour average).

O **What is the NAAQS for sulfur dioxide?**

0.03 ppm (Annual arithmetic mean for 24 hours).

O **What is the NAAQS for nitrogen dioxide?**

0.053 ppm (Annual arithmetic mean for 24 hours).

O **What is the NAAQS for carbon monoxide?**

9 ppm (8-hour) 35 ppm (1-hour).

O **What is the NAAQS for PM10?**

50 ug/m3 (Annual arithmetic mean for 24 hours).

O **One of the most important air pollution studies was the Harvard Six cities Study. Of all the factors considered, what was the most significant?**

Cigarette smoking.

O **Which criteria pollutant may act as a non-specific spasmogen in the lungs?**

Sulfur dioxide.

O **What is the major source of nitrogen oxides in our air?**

Hydrocarbon burning motor vehicles.

(O_3)

❍   **How does UV light interact with oxides of nitrogen to assist in the formation of ozone?**

UV light splits off a charged oxygen molecule, which is then free to combine with O_2 ~~for~~ to form O_3.

❍   **What other factor assist in this reaction?**

Temperature.

❍   **What season, because of these factors, has the highest ozone levels?**

Summer.

❍   **What is the water solubility of water?**

Low.

❍   **What is the water solubility of sulfur dioxide?**

High.

❍   **How does ozone contribute to respiratory illness?**

By causing release of inflammatory mediators such as cytokines.

❍   **How does ozone affect particle clearance form the tracheo-bronchial tree in humans?**

Enhances mucocillary clearance.

❍   **How does ozone affect particle clearance form the tracheo-bronchial tree in animals?**

Decreased particle clearance.

❍   **What are acid aerosols?**

When acids such as sulfur dioxide combine with particles, such as carbon.

❍   **Why are acid particles detrimental?**

They may be able to transport a relatively water insoluble substance, such as sulfur dioxide, deeper into the lung parenchyma.

❍ **What bronchoconstrictor forms from the dissociation of sulfurous acid from the hydration of SO_2?**

Bisulfite (HSO_3).

❍ **In normal subjects, what level of SO_2 is required to provoke bronchial constriction?**

Greater than 5 ppm.

❍ **In asthmatics subjects, what level of SO_2 is required to provoke bronchial constriction?**

Greater than 1 ppm.

❍ **In exercising asthmatics subjects, what level of SO_2 is required to provoke bronchial constriction?**

0.25 ppm.

❍ **Certain plants seem to thrive in sulfur rich areas of acid rain, name two?**

Wheat and rapeseed.

❍ **Nitrogen oxides are typically grouped under the name of?**

NO_x.

❍ **Following inhalation, NO_x undergoes hydration reactions to form what acids?**

Nitric (HNO_3) and Nitrous (HNO_2)

❍ **Which Pennsylvania town is famous for its deadly smog episode?**

Donora, PA in 1948.

❍ **What is the major source for carbon monoxide on earth?**

Non-anthropogenic sources such as the decay of organic mater.

❍ **Of the criteria pollutants, which is the one that is not responsible for local injury?**

Carbon monoxide.

❍ **What is the major source for large non-respirable particles?**

Erosion and abrasion, such as agriculture, and dirt roads.

WEAPONS OF MASS DESTRUCTION

○ **What are the four major nerve agents of concern today?**

Tabun, sarin, soman, VX.

○ **Which of the above four agents has the lowest LD 50?**

VX (LD50= 10 mg)

○ **Nerve agents inhibit which enzyme?**

Acetylcholinesterase.

○ **What is "aging"?**

The process whereby the bond between an organophosphate chemical and acetylcholinesterase becomes irreversible.

○ **Which nerve agent undergoes aging most quickly?**

Soman (within 2 minutes).

○ **What drug may be effective in reavtivating acetylcholinesterase prior to the completion of aging?**

Pralidoxime chloride.

○ **"GA" is the NATO designator for which nerve agent?**

Tabun.

○ **What is the NATO designator for Sarin nerve agent?**

BG.

○ **What toxin can be produced as a byproduct of caster oil production?**

Ricin.

○ **Ricin binds at what site?**

60s ribosomal subunit.

❍ **Which of the "G" nerve agents ages most rapidly?**

Soman (GD).

❍ **VX exposure can occur via which routes?**

skin, inhalation.

❍ **Which biological threat agent is caused by Coxiella burnetti?**

Q fever.

❍ **What is the causative organism for anthrax?**

Bacillus anthracis.

❍ **What is the incubation period for inhalational anthrax?**

1-6 days.

❍ **Phosgene gas exhibits an odor reminisicent of what material?**

Freshly mown hay.

❍ **What is the therapeutic end point for the administration of atropine to victims of nerve agent expsoure?**

The drying of secretions and/or ease of ventilation (not heart rate or pupil size).

❍ **What does the Mark I antidote kit consist of?**

Two autoinectors; one with 600 mg pralidoxime chloride; one with 2 mg atropine.

❍ **Which threat agent causes weakness, fever, cough, and pulmonary edema within 18-24 hours of inhalational exposure?**

Ricin.

❍ **Name the toxic product produced by intense heat applied to Teflon as found on the interior of various military vehicles:**

Perfluoroisobutylene (PFIB).

❍ **What is the antidote for exposure to the military agent known as lewisite?**

British Anti-Lewisite (BAL).

○   **What military vesicant agent is considered to be a threat agent for use by terrorists?**

Sulfur mustard.

○   **How does the treatmnet for the muscarinic effects produced by organophosphate pesticides differ from the treatment of muscarinic symptoms associated with organophosphate nerve agents?**

Atropine may be required in extremely high doses when treating organophosphate poisoning. In the face of nerve agent exposure, treatment will rarely exceed 20 mg of atropine.

○   **What is the most effective means for decontaminating individuals who have been exposed to sarin vapor only?**

Removal of clothing is all that is required.

○   **What is the most practical and effective means for skin decontamination following nerve agent exposure?**

Water.

○   **What is the NATO designator for sulfur mustard?**

HD.

○   **Following the infamous terrorist use of sarin nerve agent in the Tokyo subway what was the most common physical finding in victims of the attack?**

Miosis.

MASS-CASUALTY WEAPONS I: GENERAL, TOXINS AND RADIATION

❍ **Why is "mass-casualty weapon (MCW)" a broader term than "weapons of mass destruction (WMD)"?**

WMD implies physical destruction of property, as by explosives; mass-casualty weapons can produce large numbers of casualties without necessarily destroying property.

❍ **Give examples of mass-casualty weapons that need not be weapons of mass destruction.**

Biological agents, chemical agents, toxins, and neutron bombs (if exploded above the atmosphere).

❍ **In the setting of MCW, what is a toxin?**

A poisonous substance produced by a living organism.

❍ **Give a better term for "general poison" than "toxin."**

Toxicant.

❍ **Is a toxin a chemical agent or a biological agent?**

Although toxins are often discussed with bacteria and fungi, they are technically chemicals. They do not infect a host, they do not replicate within a host, and they are not communicable. From a clinical standpoint, they are better grouped with chemical agents or left as a separate category.

❍ **What kind of an agent is botulism?**

Botulism is technically not an agent at all; rather, it is the condition produced by the toxin formed by the bacterium *Clostridium botulinum*.

❍ **Does current U.S. doctrine permit U.S. military research and development into the offensive (as opposed to defensive) use of toxins, biological agents, or chemical agents?**

No; all research and development is for defensive purposes (e.g., medical countermeasures) only. Current doctrine prohibits even retaliatory use of these mass-casualty weapons.

❍ **Distinguish between *latent period* and *incubation period*.**

Each term describes the time between exposure to an agent and the onset of clinically observable effects; *latent period* is used for chemicals and toxins, whereas *incubation period* is used for infections caused by living organisms.

❍   **State the general relationship between latent periods and doses.**

The lengths of latent periods are generally inversely correlated to doses; that is, the larger the dose, the shorter the latent period. Knowledge of the length of the latent period can therefore often provide a valuable estimate of absorbed dose.

❍   **In what form or forms would toxins most likely to be disseminated by military troops or terrorists?**

Aerosol (an aerosol is a suspension of small particles of solids or small droplets of liquid in a gaseous medium; examples include mists, smokes, fumes, and fogs).

❍   **In what form or forms would biological agents most likely to be disseminated by military troops or terrorists?**

Aerosol.

❍   **In what form or forms would chemical agents most likely to be disseminated by military troops or terrorists?**

Solid, liquid, vapor, gas, aerosol, and combinations of these are all possibilities; the most common methods are delivery of liquids, aerosols, and gases, with associated vapor production (evaporation) from liquids, depending upon the chemical composition of the agents and depending upon environmental conditions.

❍   **What is wrong with the designation "poison gas"?**

The first chemical-warfare agents in widespread use were indeed gases and were appropriately called poison gases. As new agents such as mustard were introduced, they also came under this rubric, so that mustard, for example, became known as "mustard gas." However, mustard usually exists either as a solid (below 14° C [58° F]) or as a liquid (which may release vapor); it doesn't boil to form a true gas until it reaches 217° C [423° F])! "Nerve gas" is a similar misnomer. Thus, most chemical agents are not encountered as "poison gases."

❍   **What are the three major methods of decontaminating persons exposed to mass-casualty weapons?**

3 Chemical decontamination (using chemicals to neutralize or inactivated agents).
/ Physical decontamination (e.g., using an adsorbing agent or using water as a flushing agent).
2 Mechanical decontamination (e.g., picking or rubbing agent off the skin).

○   **What is the least important method of decontaminating exposed individuals?**

Chemical decontamination.

○   **What is the most important principle in decontaminating casualties?**

Speed; time is of the essence, at least for chemical agents, many of which begin being absorbed and begin damaging tissue within seconds to minutes of exposure even if clinical effects are delayed. The use of any decontaminating method may not remove agent that has already begun transit through the skin. The availability in several minutes of a full-body decontamination station does not relieve victims and responders from immediately removing (spot decontaminating) visible agent on the skin.

○   **What is the next most important principle in decontaminating casualties?**

Method: physical and mechanical decontamination should take precedence over chemical decontamination.

○   **What is the most effective means of applying physical or mechanical decontamination to a contaminated casualty?**

A two-step process of brief adsorption of agent by any available porous material (soil, powder, toweling, facial or toilet tissue, bread, etc.) followed by gentle removal by wiping or flushing produces the best results; if adsorbent is not at hand, proceed directly to the step of wiping, washing, or flushing. Simple rinsing with water or washing with soap and water is sufficient in most cases of skin contamination with chemical, biological, toxin, or radioactive agents.

○   **Name three important considerations to take when using water or soap and water to flush, rinse, or wash agent from the skin of casualties.**

For full-body contamination, be sure that casualties are *entirely* disrobed.
Keep shower streams and rubbing gentle; too vigorous of a shower stream or overzealous scrubbing can force contaminated material into the skin.
Pay attention to the temperature of the water and hypothermia.

○   **List disadvantages of hypochlorite solutions (bleach) for decontaminating casualties.**

Household bleach is a solution generally said to contain 5.25% hypochlorite ion, although bleach is actually a pH-dependent mixture of hypochlorous acid (HOCl) and hypochlorite ion (OCl⁻). At the alkaline pHs generally required for effective chemical decontamination, bleach is less effective as a biocide. Even at the 1:10 dilution sometimes recommended for skin decontamination, bleach can cause contact dermatitis. In alkaline solutions, it causes a liquefactive necrosis that renders the skin more permeable to the continuing absorption of chemical agents. Animal studies have shown increases in mortality in groups exposed to chemical agents and then decontaminated with bleach than in groups not decontaminated. Bleach can generate toxic byproducts from its reaction with several agents under certain conditions. Bleach gives false positives with certain chemical detectors. Bleach can act surprisingly slowly, especially against polymerized agents. Its use can give a false sense of security.

❍ **Is adsorbing, washing, rinsing, or flushing necessary in decontaminating casualties exposed solely to vapor or gas?**

Vapor and gas tend to linger in clothing and in hair (and to "off-gas" from them), but concentrations can usually be reduced to safe levels by rubbing the hair vigorously and airing clothing. Full stripping of clothing and washing of this kind of casualty will generally do no harm unless in a mass-casualty situation unnecessary full-body washing of these casualties clogs the decontamination process and delays decontamination of liquid-contaminated casualties.

❍ **What does ABCDD represent in the immediate management of a mass-casualty-weapon victim?**

Airway.
Breathing.
Circulation.
Decontamination (meaning prompt spot decontamination followed by full decontamination).
Drugs (meaning specific antidotes).

❍ **What acronym can be used to ensure that the secondary-survey assessment of a chemical or toxin casualty is thorough and does not leave out life-or-death considerations?**

ASBESTOS.

❍ **What do the letters in ASBESTOS represent?**

A: Agent(s):   Type(s) and estimated doses
S: State(s):   Solid, liquid, vapor, gas, aerosol
B: Body sites: Where exposed (routes of entry) [exposure and absorption]
E: Effects: Local vs. systemic
S: Severity: Of a) effects and b) exposure
T: Time course: Past, present, and future [prognosis])
O: Other diagnoses: a) Instead of (DDx) and b) in addition to (additional diagnoses)
S: Synergism: Interaction among multiple co-existing diagnoses

❍ **How does ASBESTOS emphasize the preventive-medicine/occupational-medicine triad of agent, environment, and host?**

The acronym starts with agent (A), follows the agent into the environment (S), investigates the passage of the agent from the environment to the host (B), assesses the interaction of the agent with the host (EST), returns to consider other possible agents (O), and then returns to the host to determine interactions of multiple agents or conditions in the host (S). This logical progression adds meaning and ease of recall to the acronym.

❍   **Why does the second S in ASBESTOS stand for both severity of effects and also severity of exposure?**

Whenever there is a latent period, there may be a disconnect between the clinical presentation of the casualty at a given point and the severity of the exposure. For example, a victim of phosgene may be only slightly short of breath three hours after exposure, but the knowledge that dose is inversely correlated to length of the latent period (T) and the knowledge that this is very short latent period for dyspnea following phosgene exposure mean that despite the fact that the clinical effects are so far only mild, the exposure is severe and will be expected to lead to progressive clinical deterioration of the casualty. Similar considerations obtain with, for example, mustard exposure.

❍   **What modifications to ASBESTOS would serve to adapt it to use with radiological casualties?**

Only the first two letters need to be reinterpreted:

A: Agent(s):   Type(s) and estimated doses (exposed, absorbed, and equivalent doses)
S: State(s):   Of matter and energy (α, β, γ, or neutron radiation)
B: Body sites: Where exposed (routes of entry) [exposure and absorption]
E: Effects: Local vs. systemic
S: Severity: Of a) effects and b) exposure
T: Time course: Past, present, and future [prognosis])
O: Other diagnoses: a) Instead of (DDx) and b) in addition to (additional diagnoses)
S: Synergism: Interaction among multiple co-existing diagnoses

❍   **Is there an equivalent acronym for the thorough assessment of casualties from biological agents?**

The acronym ARTERIOLES addresses most of the categories for each organism in the *Control of Communicable Diseases Manual*, although in a different order to reflect both a systematic progression from agent through the environment to a host and possibly from that host to other hosts:

A: Agent(s):   Type(s) of organism
R: Reservoir: Natural source (habitat)
T: Transmission: Agent to environment
E: Environment: Dispersal and persistence
R: Route(s) of entry: Body site(s) of exposure
I: Infective dose: Minimal number of organism required [potency]
O: Other hosts   Host-to-host communicability [route, period]
L: Length: Of incubation period and of clinical illness
E: Effects (clinical): Expected clinical presentation
S: Susceptibility and resistance

❍   **What is the range of aerodynamic diameters most likely to cause effects from aerosolized biological agents and toxins?**

0.5 to 5 microns (0.0005 to 0.005 mm), a range that ensures good delivery to the bronchioles and alveoli. Generally, aerosols are designed to deliver a substantial portion of particles in the range of 0.5 to 10 microns (0.0005 to 0.010 mm), since particles in this size range can remain suspended for long periods.

❍   **Define *mycotoxin*, *venom*, *endotoxin*, *enterotoxin*, and *exotoxin*.**

A mycotoxin is a toxin produced by a fungus, whereas a venom is produced by an animal. Endotoxins are lipopolysaccharide toxins in the cell walls of bacteria, and enterotoxins are toxins, such as cholera toxin, that damage intestinal mucosa. An exotoxin is a toxin that an organism releases into the environment.

❍   **What are three general mechanisms of action of toxins?**

Neurotoxicity (e.g., botulinum toxin, saxitoxin, and many venoms).
Membrane toxicity (e.g., ricin, microcystin, hemolytic snake venoms, and trichothecene mycotoxins).
Superantigen effect (e.g., staphylococcal enterotoxin B [SEB], toxic-shock-syndrome 1 [TSS-1], and streptococcal pyogenic exotoxins [SPE]).

❍   **Is there a ranking of toxins by threat?**

The Centers for Disease Control and Prevention (CDC) groups biological agents and toxins into three categories, A (the highest threat), B, and C. The categorization is available at http://www.bt.cdc.gov/Agent/agentlist.asp.

❍   **What are the toxins considered to be Category A and B agents?**

Botulinum toxin is a Category A agent; ricin, epsilon toxin from *Clostridium perfringens*, and staphylococcal enterotoxin B (SEB) are classified as Category B agents.

❍   **How many serotypes of botulinum toxin are known?**

Seven: Serotypes A through G. Types A, B, E, and F are produced from bacterial chromosomes and are the most commonly implicated in human disease; Type G comes from a plasmid, and Types C and D arise from bacteriophages.

❍   **What are the possible forms of botulism?**

Food-borne botulism, infant botulism, wound botulism, and inhalational botulism (inhalational botulism always implies toxin warfare or terrorism).

❍   **How great of a threat is waterborne botulism?**

Botulinum toxin is stable in water but is inactivated by heat (≥85° C for at least five minutes) and by chlorine (0.6 parts per million for at least five minutes). Because of dilutional effects and water treatment, botulinum contamination of public water supplies is thought not to be feasible for the production of large numbers of casualties; however, botulinum added to standing water with low chlorine residuals or to beverages could potentially be a threat.

○ **How stable is botulinum toxin in the atmosphere?**

The degradation of botulinum toxin depends upon atmospheric conditions but probably proceeds no faster than 1% to 4% per minute. Substantial inactivation (to less than 13 orders of magnitude of the original dose) would be expected by two days following release of aerosolized toxin.

○ **Can aerosolized botulinum toxin penetrate skin or mucous membranes?**

Intact skin is an effective barrier, but the toxin can be absorbed from mucous membranes.

○ **What is the mechanism of action of botulinum toxin?**

The toxin prevents the release of acetylcholine from presynaptic terminals.

○ **What are the main clinical signs of botulism?**

A one- to five-day latent period followed by progressive, descending, weakness and flaccid paralysis (with early prominent bulbar signs such as ptosis and difficulty speaking and swallowing) without fever, sensory loss, or changes in mental status. Pupillary dilatation is usually also prominent, as is drying of secretions.

○ **What was the latent period in the three known human cases of inhalation of botulinum toxin?**

About 72 hours.

○ **How important is low-grade fever as a clinical indicator of botulinum-toxin intoxication?**

Fever is not part of the typical clinical presentation of victims of botulinum toxin and should suggest the presence of a secondary bacterial infection such as aspiration pneumonia.

○ **If botulinum toxin is added to food or water, would gastrointestinal signs and symptoms such as those seen in botulism from improperly prepared or preserved food, be expected?**

Not necessarily; the gastrointestinal signs and symptoms seen in botulism from improperly prepared or stored food are thought to be related to the presence of other bacterial metabolites in the food and may not be present if purified botulinum toxin is added to food or water.

❍ **Since botulinum toxin is a motor, not a sensory, toxin, does the presence of perioral or acral paresthesias (tingling, numbness) in a suspected botulinum-toxin casualty imply another agent?**

Not necessarily; it may reflect hyperventilation from anxiety in the casualty.

❍ **What indicators in an outbreak of botulism might suggest terrorist use rather than a natural outbreak?**

Large numbers of cases with flaccid paralysis and prominent bulbar symptoms and without gastrointestinal symptoms.
Identification of an unusual type of botulinum toxin: Types, C, D, F, or G; or Type E if no aquatic source is likely.
Cases with a common geographical factor (e.g., workplace, airport, subway) but without a common dietary source.
Multiple simultaneous outbreaks without a common dietary source.

❍ **What is the usual mechanism of death in botulism?**

Respiratory paralysis.

❍ **Describe the currently FDA-approved botulinum antitoxin effective?**

It is an equine trivalent antitoxin available from the CDC and effective against Types A, B, and E, the types most commonly implicated in food-borne botulism. However, prior to administration of this antitoxin, the clinician must conduct skin testing for sensitivity to horse serum and must carry out desensitization as required.

❍ **Describe the botulinum antitoxin held by the U.S. Army.**

It is a partly despeciated equine heptavalent antitoxin (effective against Types A through G) and because of its Investigational New Drug (IND) status must be administered under informed consent. Because the risk of serum sickness is only reduced, not absent, skin testing prior to administration is recommended.

❍ **When is botulinum antitoxin effective?**

Botulinum antitoxin must be given during the latent period; it rapidly loses its effectiveness once signs and symptoms develop.

❍ **If antitoxin is not administered in time, what is the likely prognosis of a victim who has inhaled botulinum toxin?**

If ventilatory support is available, there can be gradual recovery after up to months on mechanical ventilation.

❍ **What is the source of ricin?**

The castor plant (*Ricinus communis*); together, ricin and a related agglutinin (RCA) compose 5% of the pulp from castor beans.

❍ **Name three possible routes of entry of ricin toxin into the body.**

Ingestion, injection, and inhalation.

❍ **What is the most infamous use of ricin?**

It was used in at least two attempts (one successful) at political assassination using an umbrella specially modified to inject a ricin-filled pellet.

❍ **What happens after inhalation of ricin?**

After a dose-dependent latent period of eight to 24 hours, fever, dyspnea, progressive cough, and nausea occur. Later, hypothermia and cyanosis develop; and the victim may die from diffuse necrotizing pneumonia with florid pulmonary edema.

❍ **What is the mainstay of treatment for victims who have inhaled ricin?**

Supportive, empirical therapy; no effective antidote has yet been found.

❍ **What are the three major clinical syndromes associated with the six serotypes (Types A through F) of toxins from *Clostridium perfringens*?**

Clostridial food poisoning (alpha toxin from Type A).
Clostridial myonecrosis, or gas gangrene (alpha toxin from Type A).
Enteritis necroticans, or pig-bel (alpha and beta toxins from Type C).

❍ **What is the action of epsilon toxin produced by *Clostridium perfringens*?**

Epsilon toxin, produced by Types B and D of *Clostridium perfringens*, increases capillary permeability in the intestine (thus enhancing its own absorption if ingested) and in the liver, kidney, and brain; it is associated with enterocolitis and enterotoxemia in a variety of domesticated animals and could cause damage to multiple organs in humans.

❍ **What is the significance of *Clostridium perfringens* epsilon toxin?**

It was one of the agents (along with *Bacillus anthracis* and botulinum toxin) purportedly being developed by Saddam Hussein.

❍ **What are the two main potential delivery methods for staphylococcal enterotoxin B (SEB)?**

Ingestion (leading to staphylococcal food poisoning) and inhalation (producing staphylococcal respiratory syndrome).

○ **Comment on the lethality of SEB.**

SEB was designed to produce temporary incapacitation, not death; however, high doses, especially in susceptible hosts, can be life-threatening.

○ **Briefly summarize the clinical presentation of staphylococcal food poisoning.**

Between two and eight hours after ingestion, there is sudden-onset abdominal cramping with diarrhea (usually without blood). Headache and fever may also occasionally be present. Symptoms are incapacitating but usually abate within 12 hours or less.

○ **Briefly summarize the clinical presentation of staphylococcal respiratory syndrome.**

Symptoms begin suddenly between three and 12 hours after inhalation. Fever, headache, chills, myalgias, a nonproductive cough, and dyspnea with retrosternal pain are the most prominent symptoms. Conjunctival injection may be seen from contact with aerosolized toxin, and inadvertently swallowed toxin may produce nausea and vomiting. Fever of 39-41° C (102-106° F) may persist for up to four weeks. In severe cases, death may ensue from pulmonary edema.

○ **What are ways that exposure to radiation could occur from a terrorist attack?**

Exposure could occur from the explosion of fission devices ("atomic bombs"), fusion devices ("hydrogen bombs"), enhanced radiation weapons (ERW, or "neutron bombs," which are specially modified fusion devices), radiation dispersal devices ("dirty bombs"), radiation release from a terrorist-initiated meltdown at a nuclear power plant (in this scenario, high-grade nuclear material reaches a critical mass and releases large amounts of radiation without a nuclear explosion), and clandestinely placed radiation sources.

○ **What is fallout?**

Slowly settling fine dust and debris from an explosion. In the setting of nuclear weapons, it usually refers to the radioactive debris from a fission or fusion detonation.

○ **Besides the type (fission, fusion, ERW) and yield (strength of explosion, usually in terms of tons of TNT) of nuclear weapons, what variables influence the energy production of a nuclear detonation?**

Location of the detonation. Subsurface explosions that penetrate the surface of the ground will produce large amounts of fallout, as will surface bursts, which also produce significant blast and thermal effects as well as direct radiation exposure. Airbursts at low to moderate altitudes produce little to no fallout but severe exposures to heat and radiation. Explosions at high altitudes or outside the atmosphere may produce a short but intense electromagnetic pulse (EMP) that may disrupt electronic equipment but that is not considered dangerous to human health.

❍   **What kinds of medical effects can be expected from a nuclear detonation?**

Blast (pressure) injuries, thermal injuries (burns), exposure to ionizing radiation, and psychological effects.

❍   **What kinds of blast injuries would be expected from a nuclear detonation?**

Direct injury from the shock wave ("overpressure") of the explosion and indirect injury (from victim displacement or from flying objects) associated with the extremely high-velocity winds associated with the explosion.

❍   **What kinds of burns would be expected from a nuclear detonation?**

Flash burns from direct exposure to the heat generated by the explosion, flame burns from the ignition of clothing and other flammable materials, and eyes injuries, including flashblindness (which may last several minutes) and retinal scarring.

❍   **What would be the primary mechanism of casualty production from a dirty bomb?**

Blast and heat from the conventional explosion. Severe acute illness from exposure to radiation would be unlikely, although the rates of cancers developing later on among survivors might be slightly elevated.

❍   **Distinguish between initial and residual radiation from a nuclear detonation.**

Initial radiation is predominantly composed of neutrons and gamma rays; residual radiation is that radiation still present after the initial wave of radiation from the detonation and consists of beta, gamma, and sometime alpha radiation from decaying isotopes in fallout, radioactive uranium or plutonium that did not get used up in the fission explosion, and radioactivity induced in other substances by neutrons.

❍   **Can victims of a nuclear explosion become radioactive themselves without inhaling, ingesting, or otherwise absorbing radioactive dust or other particles?**

Only if they are exposed to neutrons. Absorption of neutrons by atomic nuclei in neutron-exposed substances can produce unstable nuclei that then decay by emitting beta and gamma radiation. However, this induced radioactivity is generally seen only very close to the point of detonation (where the ground would become radioactive but where blast, heat, and initial radiation would make the likelihood of survivors minimal) or in the case of the use of an ERW ("neutron bomb").

❍   **What is the effect of radiation on casualties from toxins, chemical agents, or biological agents?**

There is a well-documented synergistic (interactive) effect between sulfur mustard and radiation, in which exposure to both radiation and mustard within a given time interval greatly increases the potency of each agent. Thus, in a combined casualty, far lower doses than usual of radiation or of mustard will suffice to cause death. Although there have been fewer studies involving the combination of radiation with other chemical agents or with toxins, it is reasonable to assume that similar interactions would occur. Radiation depresses the immune system and makes infection with biological agents far more dangerous than if no radiation injury were present.

O   **What are the three basic ways of protecting individuals against a given dose of radiation?**

Time: Decrease the time exposed to radiation.
Distance: Increase distance from the radiation source.
Shielding: Increase the shielding between the individual and the radiation source.

O   **What is the name of the constellation of signs and symptoms seen after exposure to high doses of radiation?**

Acute radiation syndrome, or ARS [see chapter on radiation].

O   **What is the role of radiation in the development of thyroid cancer?**

Radiation exposure from the atomic bombing of Hiroshima and Nagasaki, from atomic testing in the Marshall Islands, and from the release of radiation from the Chernobyl nuclear power plant has been associated with significant increases in the risk of developing thyroid cancer, especially the variant known as papillary thyroid carcinoma. Low-dose radiation given to patients to treat benign conditions such as adenotonsillar hypertrophy has also been associated with increased risk. However, low-dose radiation from diagnostic imaging studies and radiation administered either internally (for radiological ablation of the thyroid by radioiodine [I-131]) or externally (by high-dose external-beam radiation) has not been found to raise cancer risk.

O   **Is the risk of getting thyroid cancer from radiation exposure age-dependent?**

Yes; the risk is inversely related to age and may be significant for young children after exposure to even low levels of radioactive iodine. Fetuses are also presumed to be particularly sensitive.

O   **What part of the body does potassium iodide (KI) protect when given in connection with exposure to radiation?**

Only the thyroid gland.

O   **How does potassium iodide (KI) act to protect the thyroid gland from radiation?**

The thyroid normally absorbs iodine from the circulation. If some of that iodine is radioactive because of exposure of a victim to radioactive iodine released in a terrorist attack, part of the radioactive iodine will be taken up by the thyroid gland. If nonradioactive potassium iodide is administered in sufficient doses, the thyroid will tend to absorb iodine from the larger pool of nonradioactive iodine than from any circulating radioactive iodine. KI thus is said to block the uptake of radioactive iodine.

○   **Will KI protect other organs as well as the thyroid?**

No.

○   **Will KI protect the thyroid from external radiation?**

No.

○   **Will KI protect the thyroid gland from internal radiation originating from radioactive elements other than iodine?**

No.

○   **What was the main source of exposure to radioactive iodine after the release of the radioactive plume from the Chernobyl nuclear power plant?**

There was apparently little exposure to external radiation. Most of the internal radiation occurred from drinking milk from cows that had grazed in fields contaminated with radioactive iodine and, to a far lesser extent, from eating contaminated vegetables. However, the possible inhalation of radioactive iodine should still be considered to be an important risk in a terrorist incident involving radiation.

○   **During what time frame relating to exposure to radioactive iodine is KI effective?**

It may be protective even if taken three or four hours after exposure, although it should be taken before exposure or as soon after exposure as practical.

○   **How long does the protective effect of KI last?**

About 24 hours. Doses should therefore be repeated daily during the time when risk of exposure to radioactive iodine is high.

○   **What is the role of KI in protecting individuals from radioactive iodine ingested from contaminated food and drink after a terrorist release of radiation?**

Food-control measures are more important than continued KI administration. Moreover, because of the decay rate of radioactive iodine, contaminated food will pose no radiation risk once it is stored for a period of weeks or months.

○   **What is the risk to first responders and other health-care providers of radiation from external contamination of mass casualties from a terrorist event involving radiation?**

The risk is minimal. It would be extremely unlikely for any casualty to be so contaminated that he or she would pose a health risk to health-care providers from external contamination.

○ **What special protective clothing and decontamination assets are needed for radiological casualties?**

None. Water, with or without soap is sufficient to remove all contaminated material on the skin. Wounds should be flushed with saline or any other available irrigant. Bleach has no place in the external decontamination of radiologically contaminated casualties.

MASS-CASUALTY WEAPONS II: BIOLOGICAL AGENTS

○   **According to the Centers for Disease Control and Prevention (CDC), important biological diseases and agents can be grouped into three categories according to their threat potentials. How is Category A described?**

These are the highest-priority agents because they
    "a) can be easily disseminated or transmitted from person to person;
    "b) result in high mortality rates and have the potential for major public health impact;
    "c) might cause public panic and social disruption; and
    "d) require special action for public health preparedness."

    (See http://www.bt.cdc.gov/agent/agentlist.asp.)

○   **List the organisms that the CDC considers to be Category A biological agents; also list the diseases that these agents cause.**

Bacillus anthracis: anthrax.
Yersinia pestis: plague.
Smallpox virus: smallpox (*variola major*).
Francisella tularensis: tularemia.
Filoviruses (e.g., Ebola and Marburg viruses) and arenaviruses (e.g., Lassa and Machupo viruses): viral hemorrhagic fevers.

○   **Describe the kinds of agents that the CDC classifies as Category B biological agents.**

Category B agents, the second-highest-priority agents, are "a) moderately easy to disseminate; b) result in moderate morbidity rates and low mortality rates; and c) require specific enhancements of CDC's diagnostic capacity and enhanced disease surveillance."

○   **List the organisms that the CDC considers to be Category B biological agents; also list the diseases that they cause.**

Brucella species: brucellosis.
Salmonella species, *Escherichia coli* O157:H7, *Shigella*, and other food-safety threats: food poisoning.
Burkholderia mallei: glanders.
Burkholderia pseudomallei: melioidosis.
Chlamydia psittaci: psittacosis.
Coxiella burnetii: Q fever.
Rickettsia prowazekii: typhus fever.

Alphaviruses (e.g., Venezuelan-equine-encephalitis, eastern-equine-encephalitis, and western-equine-encephalitis viruses): equine encephalitides.

Vibrio cholerae, *Cryptosporidium parvum*, and other water-safety threats: Water-borne infections.

○   **What is the description of the CDC Category C for biological agents?**

These are the third-highest-priority agents and include "emerging pathogens that could be engineered for mass dissemination in the future because of

"a) availability;
"b) ease of production and dissemination; and
"c) potential for high morbidity and mortality rates and major health impact."

○   **Name two agents that the CDC considers to be Category C biological agents.**

Nipah virus and hantavirus (note that hantavirus can also be classified with viral-hemorrhagic-fever viruses).

○   **Which biological agents are the most easily transmissible from person to person through the air?**

Pneumonic plague and smallpox.

○   **What isolation precautions are applicable to healthcare workers dealing with patients who have pneumonic plague?**

Droplet precautions.

○   **What isolation precautions are applicable to healthcare workers dealing with patients who have smallpox?**

Airborne precautions.

○   **In what forms does *Bacillus anthrax* exist in the environment and in hosts?**

Bacillus anthracis can exist for decades in the soil as spores, which are also stable in water for up to two years and are chlorine-resistant; within hosts, the spores give rise to vegetative forms (active bacteria).

○   **What are the three main clinical forms of anthrax?**

Cutaneous anthrax (wool-sorters' disease, malignant pustule), gastrointestinal anthrax, and inhalational anthrax. The least common variant is oropharyngeal anthrax.

○   **Describe the main toxins produced by *Bacillus anthracis*.**

Edema toxin is composed of an A domain called edema factor (EF)—an adenylate cyclase—and a B domain called protective antigen (PA), which is a cell-binding protein. Lethal toxin is composed of an A domain referred to as lethal factor (LF)—probably a metalloprotease—and the same B domain (PA) as that found in edema toxin.

O   **Briefly describe the clinical presentation of cutaneous anthrax.**

Generally, contact of abraded skin with anthrax spores leads within several hours to a week (but usually within 48 hours) to development of a small, pruritic papule. This papule becomes a painless black ulcer with surrounding edema. The mortality in untreated and patients is 5-20% and <1%, respectively. Person-to-person transmission is rare.

O   **Briefly describe the clinical presentation of gastrointestinal anthrax.**

Acute gastroenteritis with vomiting and bloody diarrhea occurs within one to seven days after ingestion of contaminated meat. Intestinal eschars progress to generalized toxemia, and the mortality rate may be 50-100% even with aggressive treatment.

O   **Briefly describe the clinical presentation of inhalational anthrax.**

Between one day and seven days (but possibly as long as 60 days) after inhalation of anthrax spores, symptoms (sore throat, mild fever, malaise, and myalgias, and perhaps a nonproductive cough) similar to those of influenza may be seen. Later, respiratory failure and shock may ensue. Meningitis is a possible complication. The mortality rate in cases treated after clinical deterioration ensues is very high.

O   **What symptom helps to distinguish incipient anthrax from influenza-like illness (ILI)?**

Rhinorrhea is uncommon with anthrax.

O   **What general laboratory findings help to distinguish early anthrax from influenza-like illness (ILI)?**

Leukocytosis without lymphocytosis is commonly seen in early stages of anthrax; with influenza-like illnesses, WBC counts are usually low, with a relative lymphocytosis.

O   **What are the principal target tissues for inhalational anthrax?**

The lymph nodes, especially mediastinal lymph nodes; mediastinal widening from mediastinal lymphadenopathy and eventually hemorrhagic mediastinitis is a classical radiological sign of anthrax, but this finding may not be present or may be obscured.

O   **Does inhalational anthrax cause a pneumonia?**

The classical answer is no, but some cases have developed pneumonitic infiltrates.

○ **Is inhalational anthrax contagious from person to person?**

No.

○ **What is the CDC case definition for a confirmed case of anthrax?**

1. A clinically compatible case with laboratory isolation of *Bacillus anthracis* from affected tissue; or 2. A clinically compatible case with other laboratory evidence of *B. anthracis* infection based upon at least two supporting tests.

○ **What is the role of nasal swabs for those potentially exposed to anthrax via inhalation?**

Nasal swabs are useful in epidemiological studies but are neither sensitive nor specific enough to be used as diagnostic aids in individual cases. Failure to detect anthrax spores from a nasal swab does not mean that a subject has not inhaled spores, and the presence of spores in nasal passages does not necessarily mean that an infective dose has penetrated more deeply into the airways.

○ **What antibiotics are most commonly recommended as post-exposure prophylaxis for** individuals at risk of inhalational anthrax, and how long should these antibiotics be given?

Ciprofloxacillin and doxycycline; 60 days.

○ **What drug regimens have been recommended for the treatment of inhalation anthrax?**

A multidrug regimen of either ciprofloxacin or doxycycline in combination with one or more additional agents to which sensitivity testing indicates that the isolated organism is sensitive. Clindamycin has also been suggested because of its presumed antitoxin activity.

○ **How effective is the current anthrax vaccine?**

There is ample evidence to indicate that the vaccine is protective against cutaneous anthrax; its efficacy is also though to be high against inhalational anthrax, although its protection could be overwhelmed by extremely high spore challenges.

○ **How persistent is *Yersinia pestis* in the environment?**

The bacteria can live for up to a year in soil and 270 days in live tissue. It is stable in water for up to 16 days. However, most estimates are that a plague aerosol would not be dangerous after about an hour.

○ **What are the principal clinical presentations of plague?**

Bubonic plague, septicemic plague (primary or secondary), and pneumonic plague (primary or secondary).

○ **What are possible methods for military or terrorist dissemination of plague bacilli?**

Aerosol delivery and dissemination of vectors, such as the rat flea (*Xenopsylla cheopus*). (Ticks and human lice can also serve as vectors for plague).

○ **What epidemiological evidence during an outbreak of bubonic plague would suggest intentional dissemination rather than natural transmission?**

The appearance of human cases before or during, rather than after, large numbers of cases in animal reservoirs (rodents, lagomorphs, large carnivores, and domestic cats).

○ **How dangerous is inhalational plague?**

If inhalational plague is not treated within the first 24 hours after the onset of symptoms, its mortality rate approaches 100%.

○ **What is the typical incubation period for plague?**

One to seven days (longer if immunized) for bubonic plague; usually two to four days for pneumonic plague.

○ **Does pneumonic plague imply inhalational exposure?**

Not necessarily; secondary infection of the lungs can occur via hematogenous dissemination in bubonic plague.

○ **Buboes (enlarged, boggy, inflamed peripheral lymph nodes) can often be very dark in color. What is a typical difference between buboes and the black lesions of anthrax?**

Anthrax ulcers are usually painless; buboes are usually exquisitely painful.

○ **What are common signs and symptoms of pneumonic plague?**

Fever, cough productive of bloody sputum, shortness of breath, chest pain, and rapid clinical deterioration.

○ **What antibiotics have been suggested for post-exposure prophylactic therapy in asymptomatic individuals thought to have inhaled plague bacteria?**

Doxycycline (usually the first choice), tetracycline, sulfonamides, and chloramphenicol; fluoroquinolones such as ciprofloxacin have also been recommended based upon animal studies.

O   **In a contained-casualty situation involving plague victims, what antibiotic therapy is recommended?**

Parenteral streptomycin or gentamicin; chloramphenicol may be required for plague meningitis.

O   **In a mass-casualty situation involving plague victims, when IV or IM streptomycin or gentamicin is in short supply, are other antibiotic regimens suggested?**

Yes; oral doxycycline, tetracycline, or ciprofloxacin have been recommended.

O   **What was the natural reservoir for smallpox?**

Man; there was no nonhuman reservoir.

O   **Was there more than one clinical form of smallpox?**

Yes; variola major was caused by one strain of the smallpox virus, and variola minor (also called alastrim, amaas, and Cuban itch) was caused by a different strain.

O   **What were the major clinical forms of variola major?**

The typical, or classical form.
A modified, partial-immunity variant (often clinically similar to variola minor), with smaller pustules and a faster appearance and development of lesions.
Variola sine eruptione (fever without rash in some individuals with partial immunity from vaccination).
Malignant, or "flat-type," smallpox, with flat, confluent lesions and almost inevitable death.
Hemorrhagic smallpox (seen usually in pregnant women), with hemorrhages in skin and mucous membranes and a high mortality rate.

O   **What was the infection rate and the mortality rate of smallpox?**

With the usual (typical, classical form), about 30% of susceptible individuals developed disease; the mortality rate in those who did develop disease was up to 30%.

O   **What was the estimated infective dose of *Francisella tularensis* via aerosol?**

It was assumed to be about 10 to 100 virions.

O   **What is the incubation period for smallpox?**

Typically seven to 17 days, with a mean of approximately 12 to 14 days.

O   **What were the typical prodromal manifestations of smallpox, and how long did they last?**

Fever of 38-40° C (101-104° F), malaise, myalgias, and sometimes vomiting; these initial symptoms and signs usually lasted 2 to 4 days.

○ **Describe the rash of smallpox.**

The rash developed as a small maculopapular exanthem (rash on the tongue and in the mouth); by the time that these lesions ulcerated, an exanthem (skin rash) appeared beginning on the face and spreading to the trunk and extremities, including (in over 50% of cases) the palms and the soles. The exanthem was initially macular (flat) but progressed to papules and then (on about the fifth day of the rash) to vesicles that after another five days developed crusts. Pustules and scabs often co-existed for another five days; the scabs then took another six days to fall off.

○ **Contrast the rashes from smallpox (variola major) and varicella (chickenpox).**

In smallpox, the rash was synchronous (that is, most lesions were at approximately the same state of development at a given time) and *progressed* centrifugally, from the face to the extremities. The eventual *distribution* of the lesions was also said to be centrifugal, meaning in this case that there was usually a higher density on the face and distal extremities than on the trunk. In chickenpox, the rash arises asynchronously in crops after only a mild prodrome or no prodrome at all; the lesions are usually more superficial, arise first on the trunk (occasionally the face), itch intensely (smallpox lesions usually itch later, as they scab), and end up in a centripetal concentration on the trunk and proximal extremities (with or without involvement of the face and scalp) with usual sparing of the palms and soles.

○ **When was smallpox contagious?**

It was possibly contagious during the prodromal period, highly contagious during the first four days of the rash, and still contagious until the last scabs fell off.

○ **Could smallpox be transmitted by other than the respiratory route?**

Yes; transmission by fomites, although less efficient, was well-documented.

○ **When did death usually occur from smallpox?**

In the second week of the disease.

○ **Contrast variolation and smallpox vaccination.**

Variolation refers to the old practice of injecting material from smallpox crusts subcutaneously or applying the material to the surface of the skin or to the nasal mucosa; this practice usually led to a case of the modified, variola-minor-like, variant of smallpox. Vaccination against smallpox was accomplished by applying live vaccinia (cowpox) virus, which has immunological cross-reactivity with smallpox, intradermally by means of a bifurcated needle that was used to prick the skin 15 times in rapid succession. The site was then protected for a period of time to minimize the risk of autoinoculation.

❍   **When was routine vaccination against smallpox discontinued in the United States?**

Routine immunization of the general public was discontinued in 1972. Healthcare workers were no longer offered vaccination after 1976, and immunization of military recruits stopped in 1990.

❍   **What was the duration of immunity from smallpox vaccination?**

Probably about 10 years, although exposure of vaccinated individuals to smallpox after this period may result in milder forms of the disease.

❍   **What were the complications from smallpox vaccine?**

In addition to occasional autoinoculation (spread of vaccinia virus to other sites on the body of vaccine), the following complications were seen:
a) Transmission to contacts (27 per 1,000,000 vaccinations).
b) Generalized vaccinia (25 per 1,000,000 vaccinations).
c) Eczema vaccinatum (10 per 1,000,000 vaccinations).
d) Postvaccinial encephalitis (2.9 per 1,000,000 vaccinations).
e) Progressive vaccinia, or vaccinia gangrenosa (0.0 per 1,000,000 vaccinations).

❍   **On the basis of its efficacy against vaccinia (cowpox) virus, what antiviral agent has recently been suggested as possibly efficacious for post-exposure treatment of smallpox?**

Cidofovir.

❍   **What are the clinical forms of tularemia?**

Ulceroglandular, glandular, oculoglandular, oropharyngeal, pneumonic, and typhoidal (septicemic).

❍   **What would be the most likely form of tularemia to be encountered from military or terrorist use of *Francisella tularensis*?**

Pneumonic tularemia.

❍   **Can pneumonic tularemia be secondarily acquired?**

Yes; secondary pneumonic tularemia can arise via hematogenous spread in 10 to 15% of cases of ulceroglandular tularemia and in 30 to 80% of cases of typhoidal (septicemic) tularemia.

❍   **What is the estimated infective dose of *Francisella tularensis* via aerosol?**

Extremely low: about 10 to 50 organisms.

❍   **What are some clinical and radiological features of pneumonic tularemia?**

After an incubation period that is usually three to five days but that may be up to 21 days, there is usually an acute onset of nonproductive cough, dyspnea, chest pain, and pneumonia with bilateral mediastinal widening and bloody pleural effusions. Pulmonary edema may be a complication.

❍ **What is the mortality rate in untreated pneumonic tularemia?**

30 to 60%.

❍ **Is pneumonic tularemia transmissible from person to person?**

No.

❍ **What are the antibiotics of choice for most cases of tularemia?**

Parenteral streptomycin is the antibiotic of choice; gentamicin is also effective. Tetracycline and chloramphenicol are also effective, but patients treated with either of these two antibiotics exhibit significant relapse rates.

❍ **What is recommended for oral post-exposure prophylaxis of individuals exposed to *Francisella tularensis*?**

Ciprofloxacin or doxycycline.

❍ **Name one African viral hemorrhagic fever caused by an arenavirus.**

Lassa fever (from Lassa virus).

❍ **Name four South American viral hemorrhagic fevers caused by arenaviruses.**

Argentine hemorrhagic fever (from Junin virus), Bolivian hemorrhagic fever (from Machupo virus), Brazilian hemorrhagic fever (from Sabia virus), and Venezuelan hemorrhagic fever (from Guanarito virus).

❍ **Name four viral hemorrhagic fevers caused by bunyaviruses.**

Rift-valley fever (in Africa; from phlebovirus).
Congo-Crimean hemorrhagic fever (in Europe, Asia, and Africa; from nairovirus)
Hantavirus pulmonary syndrome (HPS) and hemorrhagic fever with renal syndrome (HFRS) (in Europe, Asia, and throughout the world; from hantavirus).

❍ **Name two viral hemorrhagic fevers caused by flaviviruses.**

Yellow fever and dengue fever.

❍ **What family of viruses causes Ebola and Marburg hemorrhagic fevers?**

Filoviridae (filoviruses).

❍ **What is common to the viral hemorrhagic fevers?**

Increases in capillary fragility.

❍ **How stable is the Ebola virus in aerosol form?**

It is reported to be quite stable and highly infectious, although aerosol transmission does not appear to play a significant role in naturally occurring outbreaks.

❍ **What is the most common clinical manifestation of capillary damage in viral hemorrhagic fevers?**

Flushing, petechial rashes, ecchymoses or purpura, and edema; the exception is Rift Valley Fever.

❍ **Which viral hemorrhagic fever produces exceptional edema without bleeding?**

Lassa fever.

❍ **Which viral hemorrhagic fever produces the most severe hemorrhage?**

Congo-Crimean hemorrhagic fever (CCHF).

❍ **What is the range of mortality rates in viral hemorrhagic fevers?**

From 10% in dengue fever to 90% in the Ebola-Zaire subtype of Ebola hemorrhagic fever.

❍ **Can viral hemorrhagic fevers be transmitted from person to person?**

Yes, through close personal contact, especially with infected body fluids. Contaminated syringes and needles have also transmitted cases of Ebola hemorrhagic fever and Lassa fever.

❍ **What treatment is effective for viral hemorrhagic fevers?**

Ribavirin has been successfully used in some cases of hemorrhagic fever with renal syndrome (HFRS) and Lassa fever; some patients with Argentine hemorrhagic fever have responded to the use of convalescent-phase plasma.

The international symbol to indicate a biological hazard. Although there are many variants, the color is meant to be either fluorescent orange or orange-red on whatever color background provides adequate contrast for the symbol.

MASS-CASUALTY WEAPONS III: CHEMICAL AGENTS

❍ **What three kinds of chemical compounds does the U.S. military specifically exclude from consideration as "official" chemical-warfare agents?**

Riot-control agents, herbicides, smoke and flame.

❍ **What are toxic industrial chemicals (TICs), or toxic industrial materials (TIMs)?**

Official definitions vary, but the main concept is that these are chemicals that are produced in large quantities by industrial processes and that might be used as mass-casualty weapons either on the battlefield or for terrorism. They include some common chemicals, such as chlorine and phosgene, that have also been used as chemical-warfare agents; but they also include other chemicals, generally with a toxicity equal to or greater than that of ammonia.

❍ **What does the U.S. military consider to be the two main categories of "official" chemical-warfare agents?**

Toxic agents (designed to cause death or serious injury).
Incapacitating agents (designed to cause temporary decrements in performance).

❍ **What are the four major kinds of toxic chemical-warfare agents?**

Lung agents (choking agents).
 "Blood" agents (cyanides).
Blister agents (vesicants).
Nerve agents.

❍ **What do NATO codes for chemical agents mean?**

These are one- to three-letter designations by the North Atlantic Treaty Organization (NATO) to standardize the terminology of chemical agents the common names of which may differ according to language.

❍ **Name several compounds considered by the U.S. military to be "lung agents."**

Phosgene (NATO code CG), diphosgene (DP), chloropicrin (PS), and chlorine (CL).

❍ **Name two compounds considered by the U.S. military to be "blood agents."**

Hydrogen cyanide (NATO code AC) and cyanogen chloride (CK).

○ **Name three compounds classified by the U.S. military as blister agents (vesicants).**

Sulfur mustard (NATO codes H [for impure mustard] and HD [for pure, or neat, mustard]), Lewisite (L), and phosgene oxime (CX). Phosgene oxime is actually an *urticant* rather than a vesicant, since it produces wheals (hives) rather than vesicles (blisters).

○ **Name the two main kinds of nerve agents.**

a) The so-called G agents, which were developed by Germany before and during World War II and which are watery liquids that also present a significant vapor hazard; and b) V agents, which were developed after World War II and are more viscous liquids with low volatilities.

○ **Name four G agents.**

Tabun (NATO code GA), sarin (GB), soman (GD), and cyclosarin (GF).

○ **Give the NATO code for the V agent synthesized in the United Kingdom and developed by the U.S.**

VX (referring to *o*-ethyl *S*-[2-(diisopropylamino)ethyl] methylphosphonothiolate, which has no common name).

○ **Name the anticholinergic incapacitating agent weaponized (but later demilitarized) by the U.S.**

3-Quinuclidinyl benzilate, or QNB (NATO code BZ).

○ **Name the anticholinergic incapacitating agent reputedly developed in Iraq during the 1980s and available (but not used) during the Gulf War?**

Agent 15.

○ **What are thickened agents?**

Chemical-warfare agents mixed with small amounts of a plasticizer to increase their viscosity and increase their environmental persistence; e.g., soman (GD), normally a watery liquid, can be thickened to create thickened soman, or TGD.

○ **What are "dusty agents"?**

Agents that are coated onto extremely small particles (often only a few microns in diameter) with the intent to increase agent penetration into and through protective clothing.

○ **Explain the difference between unitary and binary chemical agents.**

The difference relates not primarily to chemical composition but rather to the method of production, storage, and dissemination. Unitary agents are single chemical agents, e.g., sarin. To make binary sarin, the penultimate precursors in the chemical synthesis of sarin are stored adjacent to each other, but separated by a thin membrane, in the same container. This makes the container slightly less dangerous to store and handle. When the munition is fired, the membrane ruptures, and the precursors mix in flight to form sarin.

○ **Why do the terms "lung agents," "pulmonary agents," "choking agents," and "lung irritants" need to be used with caution if used at all?**

They are ambiguous (for example, "choking" can refer to partial or total obstruction of the larynx, trachea, or large bronchi—effects in the central airways—or to dyspnea, which is an effect in the peripheral airways) and do not specify which compartment of the respiratory tract is targeted. The military classification of "lung agents" has traditionally been used to refer to agents that damage capillaries in alveolar septa and lead to pulmonary edema, but ambiguity still exists with these terms. The CDC has included in its list of "choking/lung/pulmonary damaging" agents compounds with such diverse actions as sulfur trioxide (which predominantly affects the upper airways), phosgene (which typically targets alveolar septa), chlorine (which is intermediate in its effects), and cyanide (which is a systemic poison).

○ **What are the two important physiological divisions of the respiratory tract?**

a) The central, or conducting airways (tracheobronchial region): the portion of the respiratory tract from the larynx to about the 17th dichotomous branching of bronchioles (this is at the level of terminal bronchioles that are approximately 2 mm in diameter). This is the region in which bulk air movement occurs with each breath. Physiologically, the airways in the head and throat (nose, nasopharynx, and oropharynx) can also be added to this division.

b) The peripheral, or gas-exchange compartment: the region of the respiratory tract including the distal terminal bronchioles, the respiratory bronchioles, the alveolar ducts, and the alveolar sacs, or alveoli). This is the region in which air movement occurs only by diffusion (Brownian motion). This is because of the enormous increase in the total cross-sectional area of the airways by the time that this region is reached and the concomitant decrease in air velocity that is imposed by the constraints of a closed conduit.

○ **Is particle size a major consideration in the delivery and sites of action of chemical vapors and gases?**

No; all vapors and gases are of molecular size, and capable of penetrating all the way to the alveoli.

○ **What is a vapor?**

The gaseous state of a substance at a temperature below its boiling point at a given pressure; in other words, it is the gas that evaporates from a liquid (or sublimates from a solid) at temperatures below the temperature at which the substance boils.

❍   **What is the most common method of measuring external doses of vapors and gases that might be inhaled in a terrorist setting?**

The concentration of agent is multiplied by the duration of exposure to give the so-called concentration-time product, or Ct.

❍   **What is an LCt_{50}, and how is it related to the term LD_{50}?**

An LCt_{50} is the concentration-time product (Ct) needed to kill 50% of an exposed group. Both the LCt_{50} and the LD_{50} are measures of dose; LD_{50} implies the ability to weigh an agent and thus applies to agents in solid and liquid form, whereas LCt_{50} is used when the agent in question is encountered as a vapor or a gas.

❍   **What are the determinants of sites of action in the respiratory tract of chemical agents inhaled as vapors or gases?**

Solubility in aqueous solutions: Highly soluble gases and vapors tend to dissolve in fluids in the central compartment; less water-soluble compounds can penetrate all the way to the peripheral compartment.

Chemical reactivity: Highly chemical reactive vapors and gases tend to react with the first tissue that they encounter, that is, tissue in the central compartment of the airways. Less reactive chemicals have the opportunity to reach the peripheral compartment.

Dose: High concentration-time products of inspired vapors and gases represent such an excess that they will have effects in both the central and peripheral compartments of the respiratory tree.

❍   **When referring to inhaled chemicals, what are Type I agents?**

Agents that because of high water solubility, extreme chemical reactivity, or both, exert local effects predominantly in the central compartment of the respiratory tract in low to moderate doses. A pure Type I agent may have few to no clinical effects from systemic distribution.

❍   **When referring to inhaled chemicals, what are Type II agents?**

Agents that because of low water solubility, low chemical reactivity, or both, exert local effects predominantly in the central compartment of the respiratory tract in low to moderate doses. A pure Type II agent may have few to no clinical effects from systemic distribution.

❍   **When referring to inhaled chemicals, what are Type III agents?**

Agents that use the respiratory tract "only as an onramp to the freeway of the circulation"; that is, agents that may enter the body via inhalation but then enter the circulation, are systemically distributed to most or all the organs and tissues of the body, and exert their effects on the body as a whole.

❍   **Is the classification of inhaled agents into Type I, Type II, and Type III agents a precise classification?**

No; a more precise way of looking at the matter from a toxicological perspective would be to speak of Type I *effects* (local effects in the central compartment of the respiratory tract), Type II *effects* (local effects in the peripheral compartment of the respiratory tract), and Type III *effects* (effects on the body as a whole following inhalation and then systemic distribution). Because of the range of water solubility and chemical reactivity, few compounds are at the poles of the Type I—Type II spectrum. Also, raising the inhaled dose of almost any inhaled Type I or Type II agent will lead to effects in both compartments. Finally, many agents have local effects in one or more compartment of the lung as well as some degree of systemic toxicity. Nevertheless, grouping agents as Type I, Type II, or Type III leads to less ambiguity than referring simply to "lung agents" or "choking agents."

❍   **Name an "official" chemical-warfare agents that tends to produce Type I effects when inhaled.**

Sulfur mustard (H, HD). This agent is not very soluble in water, but its incredibly high chemical reactivity once dissolved tips the scales in favor of action in the central compartment. Sulfur mustard is, of course, officially classified as a blister agent, or vesicant; but it also acts as a Type I agent when inhaled.

❍   **Name toxic industrial chemicals that have Type I effects and that might be used as mass-casualty weapons.**

Acids such as hydrogen chloride, acetic acid, hydrogen fluoride, and sulfur dioxide; bases such as ammonia; low-molecular-weight aldehydes such as formaldehyde and acetaldehyde; acrolein (which also has Type II effects); and chloramines (which also have Type II effects). Smoke particles, although not industrial chemicals, also lodge in the central compartment of the respiratory tract and have Type I effects.

❍   **Name "official" chemical-warfare agents that tend to produce Type II effects when inhaled.**

Phosgene (CG), diphosgene (DP), and chloropicrin (PS). Chlorine (CL) is also grouped with these agents, but chlorine is intermediate both in water solubility and in chemical reactivity and exerts mixed Type I and Type II effects in almost equal proportions. Lewisite (L), a blister agent (vesicant), acts both as a Type I agent and, because of its effects on capillary permeability throughout the body, as a Type II agent in the lungs when inhaled. HC smoke, which is standard white military obscurant smoke, also has prominent Type II effects but as a smoke is officially excluded by the military from classification as an "official" chemical agent.

❍   **Name toxic industrial chemicals that have Type II effects and that might be used as mass-casualty weapons.**

Carbon tetrachloride, methyl isocyanate (the chemical released in Bhopal, India), phosgene (which is a dual-purpose chemical used extensively in industry), acrolein (which also has Type I effects), oxides of nitrogen, perfluoroisobutylene (a combustion product of polytetrafluoroethylene [Teflon]), chloramines (which have both Type I and Type II effects), and arsine (which has Type II effects in addition to its systemic effects).

○   **Name "official" chemical-warfare agents that exert Type III effects.**

The "blood" agents: Hydrogen cyanide (AC) and cyanogen chloride (CK).

○   **Name toxic industrial chemicals that exert Type III effects and that might be used as mass-casualty weapons.**

Simple asphyxiants (e.g., carbon dioxide, hydrocarbons, and oxides of nitrogen); chemical asphyxiants (e.g., carbon monoxide, hydrogen cyanide [another dual-use compound produced in large quantities industrially], hydrogen sulfide, and oxides of nitrogen); and chemicals with other mechanisms of action (e.g., arsine and stibine).

○   **What is the pathophysiology of Type I damage (damage to the central compartment)?**

a) Irritation of mucous-membranes, usually by acidic moieties released after the agent has dissolved or reacted in aqueous solution; b) Irritative laryngospasm; and c) necrosis and denudation of respiratory epithelium of conducting airways. The irritation is usually prompt; the epithelial damage may require additional time. Airways can be obstructed either by amorphous necrotic debris or by membrane-like sheets (pseudomembranes) of stripped epithelium. Necrotic debris is also an excellent culture medium for bacteria, so secondary bacterial infection is a common complication.

○   **What is the clinical hallmark of Type I damage?**

Noise! Disruption of smooth laminar flow in a conduit leads to turbulence, and turbulence creates noise. Thus, victims may cough, sneeze, become hoarse, or exhibit rales, rhonchi (wheezing), or inspiratory or expiratory stridor. Laryngospasm may also occur as a reflex reaction to irritation.

○   **What is the management of Type I airway damage?**

Provision of warm, moist, oxygenated air; bronchoscopic identification and removal of pseudomembranes as appropriate; and infection surveillance. Prophylactic administration of antibiotics is discouraged.

○   **What is the pathophysiology of Type II damage?**

Noncardiogenic pulmonary edema. Damage (usually by free radicals) to capillary endothelium in alveolar septa leads after a dose-dependent latent period, usually of several hours, to leakage of fluid into the septa, which thicken. Eventually, the hydrostatic pressure increases to the point that fluid spills into the alveoli and then tracks up the airways.

O   What is the clinical hallmark of Type II damage?

A latent period (inversely correlated with dose) followed by *dyspnea* (chest tightness, shortness of breath) without accompanying signs! The casualty may not recognize his or her actual exposure to agent. As alveolar septa thicken, it becomes harder to expand the chest during inspiration. The lungs feel, and are, stiff or tight. Dyspnea on exertion may precede dyspnea at rest. Because there is no bulk air flow in the peripheral compartment of the airway, there is no turbulence; and noise is not a component of the initial clinical presentation. Such objective evidence as end-expiratory crackles, dullness to percussion, blood-gas changes, and Kerley B lines on chest radiography are all later evidence of developing pulmonary edema.

O   When applied to a victim of a Type II agent, what does the acronym TROT represent?

Trust the patient! (Dyspnea without accompanying signs is the first clinical indicator.)
Rest the patient! (Because exertion often leads to rapid clinical deterioration, bed rest should be enforced.)
Observe the patient! (Because of the latent period, be prepared for clinical deterioration over time.)
Transport the patient! (Definitive therapy for pulmonary edema may require early transport to a pulmonary intensive-care unit.)

O   What was the classical description of the odor of phosgene?

New-mown hay, although phosgene does not smell like newly mown hay to everyone.

O   Why were Type III military chemical-warfare agents given the name "blood agents"?

The clinical effects of the first chemical-warfare agents, the pulmonary agents, were restricted to the respiratory tract; that is, they were local effects. Cyanide compounds, however, were taken up into the blood and systemically distributed; hence, these agents came to be known as "blood agents." However, all of the subsequently introduced chemical-warfare agents (vesicants, nerve agents, and incapacitating agents) can also be taken up by the blood and systemically distributed; hence, the term no longer has specificity for cyanide. Moreover, the term also suggests, wrongly, that the main site of action of these compounds is the blood. Actually, the blood serves principally as the conduit of agent from the respiratory tract to individual cells throughout the body.

O   How reliable is the smell of bitter almonds as an indicator of the presence of cyanide?

The perception of odor is extremely subjective, and what smells like almonds to one person may not smell the same to another person. Also, the sense of smell accommodates more rapidly than any of the other senses, and an initial odor may soon become undetectable because of olfactory fatigue. Most importantly, the ability to detect the characteristic odor of cyanide is conferred by a single gene that is present in only about half of the population.

❍ What is the main site of action of cyanide?

The enzyme cytochrome a_3 in the cytochrome-oxidase complex of the oxidative-phosphorylation (electron-chain, cellular-respiration) pathway in the inner membranes (cristae) of mitochondria within cells. This enzyme contains an iron atom that cycles back and forth between the 2+ oxidation state (ferrous ion) and the 3+ oxidation state (ferric ion).

❍ What is the pathophysiology of cyanide at the cellular level?

By complexing with cytochrome a_3 when it is in the ferric state, cyanide interrupts oxidative phosphorylation (cellular respiration), decreasing the energy that can be produced by the cell, preventing the cell from utilizing oxygen, and tending to the anaerobic formation of lactic acid as the cell attempts to generate energy without using oxygen. Cyanide

❍ How does cyanide exert its effect on respiration and hemodynamics?

Cyanide prevents the carotid and aortic chemoreceptors from confirming that the oxygen tension of circulating blood is in fact still normal. In cyanide poisoning, these receptors signal the respiratory center in the medulla to increase the rate and depth of breathing; the observable result is initial deep gasping. These receptors also signal the brain to instruct the adrenal medullae to release epinephrine (adrenalin) into the circulation to raise the heart rate and blood pressure; thus, tachycardia and initial hypertension are seen. The actions in the respiratory center and in the adrenal glands are attempts to increase the oxygenation of the blood and to increase oxygen delivery to tissues, respectively.

❍ Does cyanide cause cyanosis?

Not classically. The name "cyanide" is derived from the Greek *cyan*, meaning blue, only because the Prussian chemist who initially synthesized cyanide in 1782 used as his starting material ferric ferrocyanide, or Prussian blue. However, cyanide itself is colorless, and its classical clinical presentation is notable for the *absence* of cyanosis, at least in the early stages.

❍ What is the classical clinical presentation of a victim who has inhaled a large dose of cyanide?

Initial gasping, with transient tachycardia and hypertension; loss of consciousness and convulsions within about 30 seconds; convulsions; a tetanus-like presentation with opisthotonus (neck arching) and trismus (lockjaw); decerebrate posturing; bradypnea without cyanosis (in fact, the skin may appear a healthy pink); central apnea; and terminal pupillary dilatation, bradycardia, and asystole.

❍ What is the usual mechanism of death in cyanide victims?

Central apnea.

○ What are the antidotes for cyanide?

Amyl nitrite (as crushable ampoules for inhalation).
Sodium nitrite for intravenous injection.
Sodium thiosulfate for intravenous injection (immediately following the administration of the sodium nitrite).

○ Is oxygen helpful in victims of cyanide inhalation?

Because cyanide prevents the body from utilizing oxygen at the cellular level, it might seem that oxygen would not be helpful. However, oxygen has been found empirically to be useful. There is still debate over the utility of hyperbaric oxygen (HBO) in the treatment of cyanide victims.

○ Is sulfur mustard derived from the mustard plant?

No; it was called mustard because its odor was variously described as resembling that of mustard, onion, garlic, or horseradish.

○ What are nitrogen mustards?

Chemical-warfare agents similar in chemical composition (except for the inclusion of nitrogen instead of sulfur) to sulfur mustard. One, HN_2, or melphalan, became the first alkylating antineoplastic agent in medicine.

○ How irritating is sulfur mustard?

The first mustard casualties from World War I were not aware that they had been exposed and did not present for medical treatment until the following day. Humans can detect the odor of mustard at relatively low doses, but in the setting of explosions or other effects of a terrorist action, the odor may be masked or not be singled out for attention. Mustard, like phosgene and the Type II pulmonary agents, can be insidious. Mustard on the skin or in the eyes is not initially irritating.

○ Describe the absorption of sulfur mustard through skin or eyes.

Sulfur mustard is absorbed almost instantaneously through the cornea. It begins to penetrate skin almost immediately. Absorption is accelerated in skin areas that are thin, warm, moist, and oily; thus, axillae and the perineum are often involved by vapor, which penetrates clothing easily. As a dose of mustard penetrates the skin, about 10% is bound in the skin as "fixed" mustard; the remainder reaches the circulation and is systemically distributed. However, acute *clinical effects* from systemic distribution are not usually seen until lethal doses are approached.

○ What is the LD_{50} (the dose required to kill 50% of an exposed group) for sulfur mustard?

About three to seven grams (seven grams is approximately one teaspoon).

O   **What is the mechanism of action of sulfur mustard?**

Mustard dissolves very slowly in aqueous media to produce a highly active cyclic ethylene sulfonium ion that reacts with DNA, RNA, protein, cell membranes, and other cellular components. It causes both interstrand and, more importantly, intrastrand linkages in DNA.

O   **Is sulfur mustard carcinogenic?**

Yes; the International Agency for Research on Cancer (IARC) classifies sulfur mustard as a Group 1 carcinogen (carcinogenic to humans). Chronic and probably acute inhalational exposures elevate the risk of developing cancers of the nasopharynx, larynx, and lung; and chronic skin exposure elevates the risk of developing skin cancer.

O   **When does sulfur mustard start to damage tissue?**

Within the first couple of minutes. Hence, the necessity of immediate decontamination. However, if there is still mustard on the skin when the patient is first seen, even late decontamination will at least prevent absorption of the dose remaining on the skin and may prevent absorption of a lethal dose of the agent.

O   **When do mustard victims start to notice skin effects from mustard contact?**

Although fixation and damage occur within the first two minutes, the latent period for erythema and pruritus is two to 24 hours and is inversely correlated with dose. The latent period for the development of blisters is four to 36 hours. Pain is initially absent but increases as blisters develop.

O   **How dangerous is blister fluid from mustard victims?**

There is no free (unreacted) mustard in blister fluid, and blister fluid will not cause blisters.

O   **Describe the local effects of sulfur mustard on the eye.**

After a dose-dependent latent period, a chemical conjunctivitis becomes apparent, with erythema and progressive irritation and pain. Eventually the pain becomes so great that reflex blepharospasm shuts the eyes and keeps them closed. Sight is usually affected only by the fact that the victim has too much eye pain to open his or her eyes. Eye lesions usually heal over time, with photophobia that may persist over weeks.

O   **Describe the local effects of sulfur mustard on the respiratory tract.**

Because of its high chemical reactivity once dissolved, mustard acts as a Type I agent, with effects predominantly in the central compartment of the respiratory tract. However, as with any inhaled Type I or Type II agent, high doses can cause effects in both compartments, and high doses of mustard can cause pulmonary edema.

O   **Describe the systemic effects of sulfur mustard.**

Although mustard even in small doses is systemically distributed, acute clinical effects do not usually occur until the absorbed dose approaches a lethal dose. Then, mustard acts essentially as a radiomimetic agent, affecting especially cells that are dividing rapidly and cells that are poorly differentiated. The most serious effects are in the blood-forming elements of the bone marrow.

O   **What are the mechanisms of action of death in victims of sulfur mustard?**

Deaths within the first day are usually attributable either to irritative laryngospasm or to airway obstruction by amorphous necrotic respiratory epithelium or by pseudomembranes. Those who die during the next few days often succumb to a secondary bacterial pneumonia. Those who survive into the second week but who have received lethal doses experience profound bone-marrow suppression and die from septic pneumonia.

O   **What are the antidotes for sulfur mustard?**

There is no specific antidote for mustard; treatment is empirical.

O   **What toxic element does Lewisite (L) contain?**   *Antidote: BAL or dimercaprol*

Arsenic.

O   **Give three important differences between Lewisite (L) and sulfur mustard (H, HD).**

Pain after exposure to Lewisite begins within seconds to minutes.
Lewisite causes increased capillary permeability and thus a higher incidence of Type II pulmonary damage (pulmonary edema) than does sulfur mustard.
There is a Lewisite antidote: British Anti-Lewisite (BAL), or dimercaprol.

O   **What is the neurotransmitter system affected by nerve agents?**

Cholinergic transmission; that is, neurotransmission employing acetylcholine (ACh) as a neurotransmitter.

O   **Do nerve agents affect acetylcholine directly?**

No; rather, they are (anticholinesterases) which bind to and inhibit the enzyme (acetylcholinesterase, AChE) responsible for the physiological inactivation (by hydrolysis to acetate and choline) of acetylcholine after it has acted on receptors in end organs.

O   **What are the two main classes of anticholinesterases?**

Carbamates and organophosphorus compounds (often erroneously called "organophosphates" ["phosphate" implies an inorganic compound]. Nerve agents belong to the latter.

❍ **What are the differences between the actions of carbamates and organophosphorous compounds?**

Carbamates bind reversibly to AChE; organophosphorous compounds a) bind essentially irreversibly and b) set, or "age," so that after a time the agent-enzyme bond strengthens and becomes refractory to removal by oximes.

❍ **What happens in the body when nerve agents bind to acetylcholinesterase?**

The enzyme is no longer able to hydrolyze acetylcholine, which accumulates and causes two general effects on end organs: a) hyperactivity and b) fatigue and failure.

❍ **What are the clinical effects of nerve agents on the central nervous system?**

Hyperactivity results in seizures and convulsions; fatigue and failure of the respiratory center lead to central apnea.

❍ **What are the clinical effects of nerve agents on skeletal muscle?**

Hyperactivity results in twitching and fasciculations; fatigue and failure lead to weakness and flaccid paralysis, including paralysis of the diaphragm.

❍ **What are the clinical effects of nerve agents on smooth muscle?**

Miosis, bronchospasm, and hyperperistalsis (with accompanying nausea, vomiting, abdominal cramping, and diarrhea).

❍ **What are the clinical effects of nerve agents on exocrine glands?**

Hypersecretion of lacrimal, nasal, lacrimal, salivary, bronchial, digestive, and sweat glands.

❍ **How do nerve agents affect the heart?**

Although in animals nerve agents tend to induce bradycardia, the heart-rate response in humans is quite variable and includes bradycardia, normocardia, and tachycardia. The most common response in humans is actually tachycardia, but heart rate is not a reliable guide to the severity of nerve-agent poisoning.

❍ **What is the mechanism of death in nerve-agent poisoning?**

Respiratory failure, principally from central apnea, although paralysis of the muscles of respiration, bronchospasm, and bronchorrhea are contributing factors.

❍ **What are the antidotes against nerve agents?**

(antagonist of ACh)

(pry the Nerve Agent away from AChE!)

Atropine and an oxime. In the U.S., the oxime used is 2-pralidoxime chloride, or 2-PAM chloride. A benzodiazepine is also used, not for any specific antidotal effect against nerve agents but for its ability to elevate the seizure threshold.

❍ **How are atropine and 2-PAM chloride packaged for use by the U.S. military?**

As autoinjectors for intramuscular administration in the thigh through clothing. A kit composed of an atropine autoinjector and an autoinjector of 2-PAM chloride is called a MARK I kit; a new combination autoinjector containing both atropine and 2-PAM chloride is called an Antidote Treatment, Nerve Agent, Auto-injector, or ATNAA.

❍ **How does atropine work in nerve-agent poisoning?**

It acts as a competitive inhibitor of acetylcholine at postsynaptic and postjunctional muscarinic receptors in smooth muscle and exocrine glands. It can be visualized as essentially coating these receptors as the "Pepto-Bismol" of nerve-agent antidotes.

❍ **How does atropine affect twitching, fasciculations, and muscle weakness?**

These are effects of excess acetylcholine at nicotinic receptors in skeletal muscle; since atropine is an antagonist of acetylcholine essentially only at muscarinic sites, it has little to no effect on these manifestations of nerve-agent poisoning.

❍ **What are the clinical endpoints of atropine administration in a nerve-agent casualty?**

There are two: a) reduction of airway resistance and b) reduction of airway secretions.

❍ **How do oximes work in nerve-agent poisoning?**

They "pry" the nerve agent away from acetylcholinesterase; hence, the nickname "2-PAM crowbar" for 2-PAM chloride.

❍ **What are the clinical effects of oximes when used in nerve-agent poisoning?**

Clinically, oximes tend to decrease twitching and fasciculations and restore muscle strength; they are thus clinically complementary to atropine.

❍ **What are two caveats in the administration of oximes in nerve-agent poisoning?**

a) Because of the possibility of adverse side effects, including possible hypertension, repeat doses via autoinjectors should be spaced an hour apart after the first three injections and b) oxime administration is ineffective after aging of the nerve agent with acetylcholinesterase occurs. In practical terms, this is a problem only with soman (GD), nearly all of which has aged after about ten minutes. With the other G agents and with VX, aging occurs over a period of hours to days, and oximes will be effective during this time.

○ **What role does cholinesterase testing have in the acute management of nerve-agent casualties?**

None. Cholinesterase activity is useful in an occupational setting with workers at risk of exposure. It may also help to monitor convalescence. However, nerve-agent poisoning is an emergency that is acutely managed on a clinical, empirical basis.

○ **What is 3-quinuclidinyl benzilate (QNB, NATO code BZ)?**

An anticholinergic glycolate that was initially developed as a medication against postoperative nausea and vomiting but because of the prominent side effect of confusion was never marketed for this use. Instead, it was developed and stockpiled by the military forces of the U.S. and several other countries for potential battlefield use as an incapacitating agent. Destruction of U.S. stockpiles of this agent began in 1988 and is complete.

○ **What is the safety ratio of BZ?**

The ICt_{50} (the concentration-time product needed to produce incapacitation in 50% of an exposed group) is about 110 mg-min/m^3, whereas the LCt_{50} (the concentration-time product expected to kill half of an exposed group) is about 200,000 mg-min/m^3. Thus, the safety ratio for BZ is approximately 2,000. Deaths may nevertheless occur from a) overwhelming dose, b) untreated heat stress, or c) hallucination-impelled irrational acts.

○ **What is Agent 15?**

The name given to the anticholinergic glycolate stockpiled by Saddam Hussein prior to the Gulf War.

○ **What nerve-agent antidote is also an anticholinergic glycolate?**

Atropine.

○ **What is the mechanism of action of anticholinergic glycolates?**

They act as competitive inhibitors of acetylcholine at muscarinic sites both in the peripheral nervous system (PNS) and in the central nervous system (CNS). This is the basis of the use of atropine against the cholinergic crisis induced by nerve agents. However, when anticholinergic compounds are administered to an individual who has the normal amount of acetylcholine, acetylcholine deficiency ensues.

○ **Why isn't atropine classed as an incapacitating agent?**

Atropine in large doses can produce confusion. However, BZ is far more potent in this regard.

❍ **What are the effects of anticholinergic incapacitating agents in the peripheral nervous system (PNS)?**

Because of blockage of acetylcholine at postjunctional muscarinic receptors in the pupillary constrictor musculature of the eye, the normal tone of the noradrenergically innervated pupillary dilator muscle is unopposed, and mydriasis (pupillary dilatation) results. This and the associated paralysis of accommodation make vision blurred.

Because of lack of cholinergic stimulation at muscarinic receptors in exocrine glands, secretions are reduced.

Because of anhidrosis, core temperature rises.

Because of efforts to dissipate heat by opening arteriovenous shunts in superficial blood vessels in the dermis, the skin appears flushed (the so-called "atropine flush" when seen with atropine).

Because of lack of stimulation of muscarinic receptors in smooth muscle, bowel sounds may be absent and there may be constipation.

❍ **What is the classical way of summarizing the first four of the PNS elements of the anticholinergic toxidrome?**

The patient is a) "blind as a bat," b) "dry as a bone," c) "hot as a hare," and d) "red as a beet."

❍ **What are the effects of BZ in the central nervous system (CNS)?**

BZ causes lethargy progressing through stupor through coma, disturbances in judgment and insight, disorientation, ataxia, and so-called "phantom behaviors" (disrobing and picking at imaginary objects ["woolgathering"] in addition to illusions and hallucinations.

❍ **Contrast BZ-induced hallucinations to hallucinations induced by psychedelic indoles such as LSD.**

Psychedelic hallucinations tend to be abstract, geometric, and ineffable (difficult to describe). Synesthesia (sensory crossover) may also be seen. Anticholinergic hallucinations tend to be concrete and to decrease in size over time (they are sometimes called "Lilliputian" hallucinations). There may be social sharing of illusions and hallucinations (*"folie à deux,"* *"folie en famille,"*).

❍ **What is the classical way of summarizing the CNS component of the anticholinergic toxidrome?**

The patient is "mad as a hatter." However, this phrase arose not in the milieu of anticholinergic poisoning but rather as a reference to abnormal behavior in hatters, supposedly from mercury intoxication (the real contribution of mercury is still being debated).

○   **Is there a specific antidote for BZ?**

Physostigmine, a nonpolar carbamates anticholinesterase, penetrates the blood-brain barrier and binds reversibly to acetylcholinesterase, thus decreasing the ability of this enzyme to hydrolyze acetylcholine and temporarily increasing the concentration of acetylcholine at postsynaptic muscarinic receptors in the brain. However, because it has nerve-agent-like effects (including apnea and seizures) in overdosage and can even induce hallucinations (!), it should be used with caution. It may often not been needed. It is also important to recognize that because physostigmine is a reversible anticholinesterase it does not shorten the clinical course (which may last several days) of anticholinergic poisoning, and periodic redosing or establishment of an intravenous infusion may be necessary.

○   **What are the other mainstays of management of a BZ victim?**

Removal of dangerous items, restraint, reassurance, management of heat stress (from anhidrosis), and evacuation.

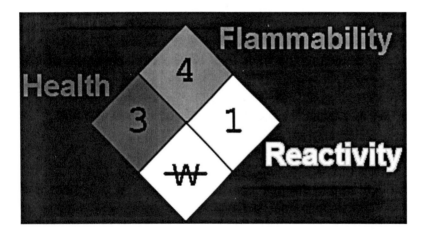

The National Fire Protection Agency (NFPA) symbol for chemical hazards. Chemical-warfare agents would all have a 4 (the number representing the highest threat) in the small health diamond of the large diamond.

BIBLIOGRAPHY

The 5 Minute Emergency Medicine Consult, Rosen, Peter; Barkin, Roger M.; Hayden, Stephen R.; Schaider, Jeffrey J.; Wolfe, Richard, Lippincott Williams & Wilkins (2003)

Atlas Of Emergency Medicine, Knoop, Kevin J., McGraw-Hill Professional Publishing, (August 2001)

Atlas Of Pediatric Emergency Medicine, Shah, Binita R., McGraw-Hill Publishing Co (January 2004)

Cancer as an Environmental Disease, nicolopoulou-Stamati, Kluwer Academic Publishers, 2004.

Clinical Practice Of Emergency Medicine, Harwood-Nuss, Ann (Edt); Wolfson, Allan B., Md (Edt); Linden, Christopher H., Md (Edt); Shepherd, Suzanne Moore, Md (Edt); Stenklyft, Phyllis Hendry, Md (Edt), Lippincott Williams & Wilkins, (December 2000)

Clinical Procedures In Emergency Medicine, Roberts, James R., Elsevier - Health Sciences Division (January 2003)

Emergency Medicine, Tintinalli, Judith E., McGraw-Hill Companies (September 2003)

Emergency Medicine, Ma, O. John, McGraw-Hill Publishing Co (January 2004)

Emergency Medicine Manual, John, Ma O., McGraw-Hill Publishing Co, (January 2003)

Emergency Medicine On Call, Keim, Samuel, Lange Medical Books/McGraw-Hill Medical Pub. (January 2003)

Emergency Medicine Secrets, Markovchick, Vincent J., Lippincott Williams & Wilkins, (January 2002)

Emergency Medicine: Concepts And Clinical Practice. 3 Volume Set, Rosen, P., Elsevier Science Health Science Div (2002)

Environmental Health, Hilgenkamp, Kathryn, Jones & Bartlett, 2004.

Environmental Health, Moeller, Dade, Harvard University Press, 2004.

Field Guide to Wilderness Medicine, Auerback, Paul, Elsevier, Science, 2003.

Geriatric Emergency Medicine, Meldon, Stephen, McGraw-Hill Professional Publishing (January 2003)

Occupational Health, Acutt, Jenny, Juta 7 Company, 2004.

Occupational and Environmental Neurotoxicology, Feldman, Robert, Lippincott Williams & Wilkins, 1998.

Occupational and Environmental Medicine, McCunney, Robert, Lippincott Williams & Wilkins, 2004.

Osha Occupational Radiation Safety, Farb, Daniel, 2003.

Ticks and What You Can Do About Them, Drummond, Roger, Wilderness Press, 2004.

Wilderness Medicine, Auerbach, Paul, Elsevier Science, 2001.

CPSIA information can be obtained at www.ICGtesting.com
Printed in the USA
LVOW09s1604020813

345735LV00003B/80/P